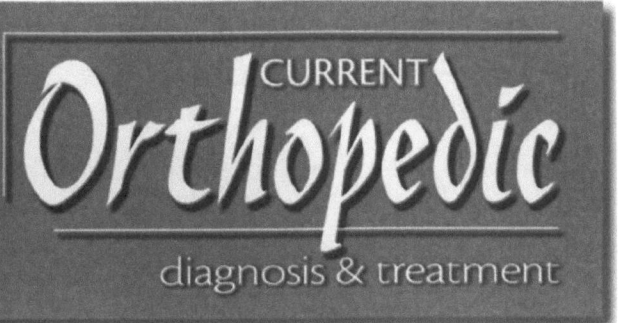

CURRENT
Orthopedic
diagnosis & treatment

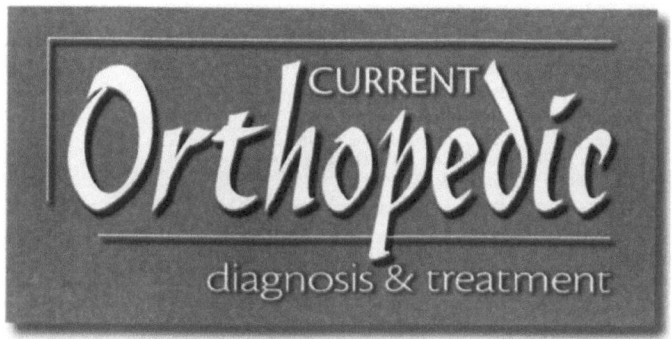

Edited by

James D. Heckman, MD

Professor and Chairman
Department of Orthopedics
University of Texas Health Science Center
San Antonio, Texas

Robert C. Schenck, Jr., MD

Professor
Department of Orthopedics
University of Texas Health Science Center
San Antonio, Texas

Animesh Agarwal, MD

Assistant Professor
Department of Orthopedics
University of Texas Health Science Center
San Antonio, Texas

Current Medicine, Inc.
Philadelphia

Current Medicine, Inc.

400 Market Street
Suite 700
Philadelphia, PA 19106

Managing Editor	Mary Kinsella
Editorial Supervisor	Jennifer Wood
Developmental Editor	Marilyn J. Bess
Editorial Assistant	Forrest Rian Perry
Art Director	Jerilyn Kauffman
Layout	Erika Mangan, Rachel Berlin, and Christy Keller-Quirk
Illustration Director	Debra Wertz
Illustrator	Wieslawa Langenfeld
Cover Design	Erika Mangan
Production Manager	Lori Holland
Production Associate	Peter O'Steen
Indexing	Dorothy Hoffman

Library of Congress Cataloging-in-Publication Data

Current orthopedic diagnosis and treatment / edited by James D. Heckman ; developed by Current Medicine, Inc.
    p. ; cm.
    Includes bibliographical references and index.
    ISBN-13:978-1-57340-141-8   e-ISBN-13:978-1-4613-1107-2
    DOI: 10.1007/978-1-4613-1107-2

    1. Orthopedics—Handbooks, manuals, etc. I. Title: Orthopedic diagnosis and treatment. II. Heckman, James D. III. Current Medicine, Inc.
    [DNLM: 1. Musculoskeletal Diseases—diagnosis—Handbooks. 2. Musculoskeletal Diseases—therapy—Handbooks. 3. Musculoskeletal System—injuries—Handbooks. 4. Orthopedic Procedures—Handbooks. WM 39 C976 1999]
    RD731.C865 1999
    616.7—dc21
                                                                    99-044555

For more information please call 1-800-427-1796 or
e-mail us at inquiry@phl.cursci.com
www.current-sciencegroup.com

ISBN-13:978-1-57340-141-8

5 4 3 2 1

It is with a great deal of pleasure that the Department of Orthopedics at the University of Texas Health Science Center at San Antonio offers this contemporary review of common musculoskeletal conditions for all physicians. It is our hope that the most common of musculoskeletal conditions will be presented in a way that is clear and concise to facilitate both the diagnosis and the specific treatment. Virtually the entire faculty of the Department of Orthopedics participated in this project, but I give special thanks to Robert C. Schenck, Jr., MD and to Animesh Agarwal, MD for the tremendous amount of time that they spent editing and facilitating the processing of the manuscripts. Special thanks should be given also to Anne Little, who served as a copy editor and organizer for the project. We all hope that the ideas presented here will benefit clinicians' practices and how they treat their patients.

James D. Heckman

Robert M. Campbell Jr., MD
Department of Orthopedics
University of Texas Health Sciences Center
San Antonio, Texas

Fred G. Corley, MD
Professor
Department of Orthopedics
University of Texas Health Sciences Center
San Antonio, Texas

Philip Jacobs, MD
Clinical Assistant Professor
Department of Orthopedics
University of Texas Health Sciences Center
Orthopedic Surgeon
Orthopedic Surgery Associates of San Antonio
San Antonio, Texas

Jay D. Mabrey, MD
Associate Professor
Department of Orthopedics
University of Texas Health Sciences Center
San Antonio, Texas

Peter L.J. McGanity, MD
Professor
Department of Orthopedics
University of Texas Health Sciences Center
Orthopedic Attending Surgeon
University Hospital/University Health System
San Antonio, Texas

Robert Ward, MD
Department of Orthopedic Surgery
University of Alabama School of Medicine
Birmingham, Alabama
Administrative Chief Resident
Department of Orthopedics
University of Texas Health Sciences Center
San Antonio, Texas

Jeffrey R. Warman, MD
Clinical Assistant Professor
Department of Orthopedics
University of Texas Health Sciences Center
Orthopedic Surgeon
Pediatric Orthopedic Associates
San Antonio, Texas

Michael A. Wirth, MD
Associate Professor
Department of Orthopedics
University of Texas Health Sciences Center
Chief
Orthopedic Shoulder Service
Audie Murphy Veterans Hospital
San Antonio, Texas

CONTENTS

CONTENTS

CONTENTS BY SPECIALTY

CONTENTS BY SPECIALTY

This book provides current expert recommendations on the diagnosis and treatment of all major disorders throughout orthopedics in the form of tabular summaries. Essential guidelines on each of the topics have been condensed into two pages of vital information, summarizing the main procedures in diagnosis and management of each disorder, to provide a quick and easy reference.

Each disorder is presented as a "spread" of two facing pages: the main procedures in diagnosis on the left and treatment options on the right.

Listed in the main column of the Diagnosis page are the common history, physical findings, and complications of the disorder, with brief notes explaining their significance and probability of occurrence, together with details of imaging and laboratory studies that can be used to aid diagnosis.

The **left shaded side column** contains information to help the reader evaluate the probability that an individual patient has the disorder. It may also include other information that could be useful in making a diagnosis (eg, classification or grading systems, comparison of different diagnostic methods).

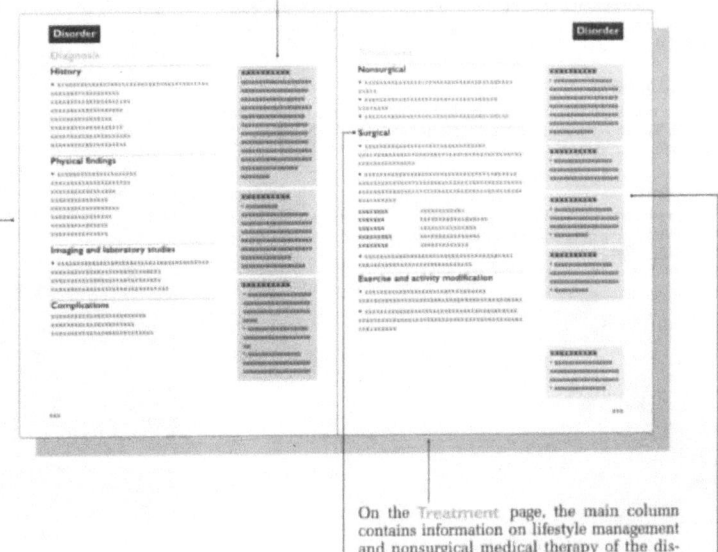

On the Treatment page, the main column contains information on lifestyle management and nonsurgical medical therapy of the disorder, with general information on surgical management when this is the main treatment.

Whenever surgery is necessary, "Surgical treatment" gives indications for the proper types of surgery and their uses. Efficacy, risk assessment, and cost–benefit analysis of specific surgical procedures are discussed as appropriate. This section provides additional information about perioperative care and other surgical concerns.

The main goals of treatment (eg, to cure, to palliate, to prevent), prognosis after treatment, precautions that the physician should take during and after treatment, and any other information that could help the clinician to make treatment decisions (eg, other nonpharmacologic treatment options, special situations or groups of patients) are given in the **right shaded side column**. The key and general references at the end of this column provide the reader with further practical information.

1

J.D. Heckman

Diagnosis

History

Achilles tendon rupture usually occurs in athletic individuals in their early middle-age years. Sometimes there is a prodromal period of pain and swelling in the area of the Achilles tendon, but often the patient is not symptomatic before the injury. The injury typically occurs during racquet sports or basketball as the player suddenly reaches toward the ball and acutely dorsiflexes the foot, stretching the Achilles tendon. Often, a loud snap is heard as the tendon ruptures. Pain and swelling immediately occur, but some plantarflexion power remains because the posterior tibial and peroneal musculotendinous units remain intact.

Physical findings

Swelling and perhaps ecchymosis in the distal posterior calf develop immediately after the injury. On palpation the course of the Achilles tendon is tender, and a defect in the tendon can sometimes be palpated an inch or two above the tuberosity of the calcaneus. Plantarflexion power is weak, and usually the patient cannot stand on tiptoes. Thompson's test is performed by having the patient lie prone with the foot hanging over the edge of the table while the examiner squeezes the calf manually. When the Achilles tendon is ruptured, the foot will not passively plantarflex as it does if the tendon is intact.

Imaging and laboratory studies

Radiographs are usually normal. Ultrasonography can be used to demonstrate the defect in the Achilles tendon, but the diagnosis can be made simply on physical examination.

Complications

Failure to diagnose an acute Achilles tendon rupture leads to contracture of the muscle and a persistent gap between the ruptured tendon ends. Plantar flexion power will remain weak.

Differential diagnosis

An acute dorsiflexion force applied to the ankle can sometimes cause isolated rupture of the medial head of the gastrocnemius muscle. This is a much more benign condition that heals well without aggressive treatment. In this injury, the Achilles tendon remains intact and long-term function is excellent. Sometimes it is difficult to distinguish these two conditions if the patient's calf is swollen and diffusely tender.

Etiology or pathophysiology

Middle-aged adults are particularly prone to Achilles tendon rupture because the Achilles tendon often undergoes degenerative changes (tendinosis) during the aging process. As a result, it can no longer withstand vigorous athletic activity.

Epidemiology

Achilles tendon rupture usually occurs in men in their early middle-aged years. Frequently the men are "weekend warriors" who sustain the injury while playing tennis or basketball.

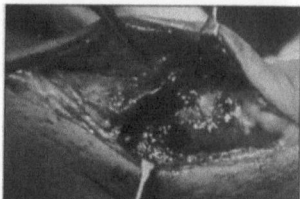

Figure 1. An acute rupture of the achilles tendon in midsubstance.

Treatment

Nonsurgical

Holding the ankle and foot passively in a plantarflexed posture for 8 to 9 weeks allows the torn tendon ends to lie in close approximation within the tendon sheath, where they can heal together with scar tissue. This healing is not as secure as that provided by surgical repair, and approximately 10% of patients who are treated by such closed means in a cast will rupture the tendon again when they resume vigorous activity. Thus, nonsurgical treatment is usually reserved for older patients with a more sedentary lifestyle.

Surgical

Surgical repair of the acutely torn Achilles tendon is relatively easy. The frayed tendon ends are exposed directly and are sutured together with two or three heavy, nonabsorbable sutures. After surgery, the foot must be held in a slightly plantarflexed posture in a cast or a functional brace for 6 to 8 weeks to allow full healing. Surgical repair is sometimes complicated by wound infection, breakdown, and slough of the repaired Achilles tendon, creating a large defect that is difficult to reconstruct.

Exercise and activity modification

Because middle-aged adults are particularly prone to this injury when participating in athletic activities, they should conscientiously participate in a vigorous heelcord stretching program on a daily basis and focus on heelcord stretching before participating in athletic activities.

Treatment aims

To restore the integrity of the Achilles tendon and the normal length of the musculotendinous unit. If the musculotendinous unit heals in a lengthened position, plantarflexion power will be persistently weak, creating a limp and the inability to run and jump vigorously.

Prognosis

The prognosis for recovery is excellent if repair is prompt. Delay in diagnosis leading to contracture of the muscle creates a difficult reconstructive problem for the surgeon. Often, patients with a chronic tear of the Achilles tendon have persistent weakness and limited function.

Follow-up and management

Immobilization for 6 to 9 weeks is necessary after surgical repair or closed treatment of the ruptured Achilles tendon. During this period, the patient must remain on crutches and should not bear weight on the affected side. Once the repair is healed, rehabilitation is pursued with 2 to 3 months of strengthening and range-of-motion exercises for the ankle.

Key references

1. Seltzman and Tearse: Achilles tendon injuries. *J Am Acad Orthop Surg* 1998, 6:316–325.

2. Acetti R, Henriksen LO, Jacobson KS: A new treatment of ruptured Achilles tendons: a prospective randomized study. *Clin Orthop* 1994, 308:155–165.

Diagnosis

History

The most common cause of acromioclavicular joint injury is a direct blow that occurs when the patient falls onto the point of the shoulder.

Physical findings

Mild to moderate discomfort and swelling occurs with incomplete acromioclavicular joint injuries (Types I and II, in which the capsular ligaments are strained or torn but the coracoclavicular ligaments remain intact). Patients with complete dislocations of the acromioclavicular joint (Types III to VI, in which the capsular and coracoclavicular ligaments are torn) characteristically present with the arm held close to the body and supported in an elevated position to relieve pain at the joint. The distal clavicle is usually prominent and markedly tender to palpation (Fig. 1). Any motion, especially elevation, increases pain.

Complications

Neurologic insult, such as a brachial plexus neuropraxia, is uncommon but may occur early or late after acromioclavicular joint dislocations.

Residual deformity is common and may be cosmetically unacceptable to some patients.

Skin ulceration may occur over the acromioclavicular joint secondary to the immobilization device.

Pain and fatigue may occur in overhead laborers with complete acromioclavicular joint injuries that are not stabilized surgically.

Differential diagnosis

Glenohumeral dislocation, clavicle fracture, acromial or coracoid fracture, or osteolysis of the distal clavicle.

Etiology or pathophysiology

Acromioclavicular joint injuries represent a spectrum ranging from strain of the capsular ligaments to complete disruption of the capsular and coracoclavicular ligaments. Although there may be slight upward displacement of the clavicle by the pull of the trapezius muscle, the true anatomic feature is downward displacement of the upper extremity.

Epidemiology

Acromioclavicular joint injuries are among the most common sports injuries of the shoulder (Fig. 2). The incidence of incomplete to complete acromioclavicular joint dislocations is approximately 2:1 and most involve male patients.

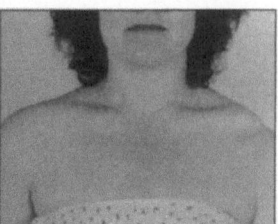

Figure 2. Patient with a complete acromioclavicular joint dislocation of the left shoulder.

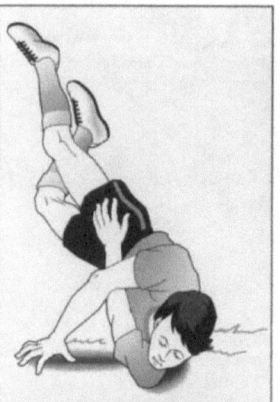

Figure 1. An acromioclavicular injury most commonly is the result of a fall on the shoulder.

Treatment

Nonsurgical

Most injuries (Types I to III) are managed with ice for the first 12 to 24 hours and a sling until symptoms improve. Activities are increased as tolerated. Heavy lifting and contact sports are delayed until the patient has full range of motion and minimal to no pain (usually 4 weeks).

Surgical

Surgery is recommended primarily for patients with Type III injuries who perform heavy labor and for all patients with Type IV to VI injuries because of the degree of soft tissue injury and the severe amount of distal clavicle displacement. Surgical technique involves coracoclavicular ligament repair and restoration of the vertical and horizontal stability of the acromioclavicular joint by means of a temporary coracoclavicular lag screw.

Treatment aims

To reduce swelling and pain so that the patient may resume preinjury work and sports.

Prognosis

Motion and strength return within 3 to 6 weeks.
Overhead heavy laborers may experience discomfort and fatigue if not injury is not repaired surgically.

Follow-up and management (or rehabilitation)

Sling for 2 weeks.
Patient encouraged to perform simple activities of daily living.
Patient instructed to avoid lifting, pushing, and pulling for 6 weeks.
Routine screw removal at 6 to 8 weeks.

Key references

1. Guy DK, Wirth MA, Griffin JL, et al.: Reconstruction of chronic and complete dislocations of the acromioclavicular joint. *Clin Orthop Rel Res* 1998, 347:138–149.
2. *Fractures* edn 2. Edited by Rockwood CA Jr, Green DP. Philadelphia: JB Lippincott; 1984.
3. Wirth MA, Rockwood CA Jr.: *Operative Orthopaedics*, edn 2. Edited by Chapman MA, Madison M. Philadelphia: JB Lippincott; 1993.

Diagnosis

History

Adult acquired flatfoot is associated with pain, swelling along the medial aspect of the ankle and the arch of the foot, and gradual collapse of the longitudinal arch of the foot with weight bearing. Rarely is there a history of injury. The pain is aggravated by standing and walking and is relieved by non–weight-bearing and nonsteroidal anti-inflammatory drugs. With the chronic form of this condition, patients also develop lateral midfoot pain as the calcaneus impinges on the distal fibula.

Physical findings

Swelling and sometimes redness along the medial aspect of the ankle extends into the arch of the foot. With weight bearing, the longitudinal arch of the foot collapses; when viewed from behind, there is a "too many toes" sign (more toes are seen on the lateral side of the affected foot than on the unaffected foot). Often, the patient cannot raise on tiptoe on the affected side. Manual muscle testing shows limited active inversion of the heel, which is consistent with impaired function of the posterior tibial musculotendinous unit. The course of the posterior tibial tendon (from the musculotendinous junction behind the medial malleolus to the tendon's insertion on the navicular tuberosity) is markedly tender to palpation.

Imaging and laboratory studies

Standing anteroposterior radiographs of the foot show collapse of the longitudinal arch, with a prominent sag at the talonavicular joint.

Complications

Chronic and persistent stretching of the posterior tibial tendon leads to inflammation and eventual rupture.

Differential diagnosis
Arthritis of the subtalar and midtarsal joints.

Etiology or pathophysiology
The cause of adult-acquired flatfoot is not clearly understood. Some investigators feel that the underlying abnormality is a stretch or tear of the spring (calcaneonavicular) ligament that normally supports the head of the talus and prevents it from rolling into the arch of the foot with weight bearing. As the ligament stretches or tears, a greater demand is placed on the posterior tibial musculotendinous unit to provide dynamic support for the longitudinal arch. The tendon then becomes inflamed and painful and may eventually rupture. Chronic collapse of the arch of the foot creates stress on the rearfoot, leading to degenerative arthritis of the subtalar and midtarsal joints.

Epidemiology
This condition usually occurs in middle-aged or elderly women.

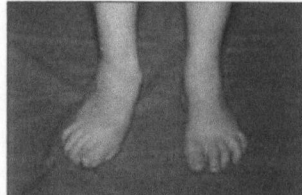

Figure 1. A patient with adult acquired flatfoot on the right side. Note flattening of the arch and lateral deviation of the toes.

Treatment

Nonsurgical

In the early phases of this disorder, aggressive nonsurgical treatment may short-circuit the problem. Cast immobilization lasting 4 to 6 weeks allows the acute inflammation to subside; the foot should then be supported with a custom-molded University of California Berkeley Laboratories (UCBL) orthosis, which can be fitted into an Oxford-type shoe. This insert supports the longitudinal arch, controls the subtalar joint, and protects the chronically inflamed posterior tibial tendon. Nonsteroidal anti-inflammatory drugs help to decrease the inflammation in and around the tendon, and a physical therapy program that includes strengthening of the posterior tibial tendon and heel-cord stretching helps to restore function.

Surgical

A variety of surgical procedures to treat this condition have been described. Acute inflammation of the posterior tibial tendon should be treated with aggressive debridement of the inflamed synovium and removal of any frayed tendon ends. Disruption of the spring ligament complex should be repaired primarily, and a completely torn or extensively scarred posterior tibial tendon should be reconstructed using the flexor digitorum communis as a tendon transfer. In chronic cases, tendon decompression or reconstruction alone is usually insufficient and should be combined with subtalar, talonavicular, or triple arthrodesis to permanently restore the integrity of the longitudinal arch.

Exercise and activity modification

Because the condition is aggravated by prolonged standing and walking, these activities should be avoided. The foot should be supported and protected in a shoe with a substantial longitudinal arch support.

Treatment aims
The initial goal is to relieve pain, swelling, and inflammation of the posterior tibial tendon. Aggressive treatment should be pursued to prevent rupture of the tendon. Chronic acquired flatfoot deformity requires treatment with stabilization of some or all of the rearfoot joints to restore the longitudinal arch.

Prognosis
Once established, this condition is often recalcitrant. It is not uncommon for the patient to have some persistent, residual, long-term flattening of the longitudinal arch and symptoms of rearfoot arthritis as a consequence of the condition.

Follow-up and management
When the condition is stabilized, use of proper shoewear (an Oxford shoe with a longitudinal arch support) is required. Gradual resumption of moderate physical activities can be anticipated, but returning to vigorous running and jumping probably will be difficult, if not impossible.

Key references
1. Myerson MS: Adult acquired flatfoot deformity. *J Bone Joint Surg* 1996, 78:780–792.

Diagnosis

History

Most patients who sustain ankle fractures usually report "twisting" their ankle. The injury is usually of the inversion type, although many mechanisms can occur. The patient usually reports immediate inability to bear weight and swelling. Some, however, may have walked on the ankle for days before presentation if the fracture is nondisplaced or is in a stable pattern. Ankle fractures are also caused by high-energy injuries. These usually result in open or comminuted fracture patterns and make treatment options challenging.

Physical findings

Mild to severe ankle swelling depends on the treatment instituted by the patient immediately after injury and the time from injury to presentation. The patient usually has exquisite tenderness to palpation directly over the bone. Crepitus may be present. The patient experiences pain when attempting to bear weight. Depending on the severity of the injury, the patient also may have significant instability. Range of motion is limited and is usually related to pain or instability. An associated finding of tibiotalar dislocation or subluxation may be present (Fig. 1). It is important to assess the neurovascular status of the foot, especially in open fractures.

Imaging and laboratory studies

Standard radiographs include the anteroposterior, lateral, and mortise views. Recently, however, the use of anteroposterior radiographs in the treatment of ankle fractures has been questioned. Computed tomography is not indicated in routine management of ankle fractures unless significant joint involvement is present (making the fracture behave more like a tibial pilon fracture). Magnetic resonance imaging is also rarely indicated, although it has been useful in assessments for associated osteochondral lesions of the talus in patients who are in chronic pain after treatment of ankle fracture.

Complications

Failure to diagnose an unstable ankle fracture can lead to associated posttraumatic instability and arthritis. Fortunately, most fractures are diagnosed within several days of injury, and in most cases delayed diagnosis is due to delayed presentation. Diagnosis may be delayed in trauma patients because of the focus on associated life- and limb-threatening injuries. All patients develop some stiffness after cast removal or after postoperative treatment. Significant calf atrophy can also be disabling. With proper anatomic restoration of the ankle mortise, posttraumatic arthritis is not a problem. Other complications with surgical treatment are infection, hardware failure, and hardware pain or prominence requiring plate and screw removal.

Differential diagnosis

An ankle fracture must be differentiated from a simple ankle sprain. Infection, Charcot arthropathy, tibial pilon fracture, and tibiotalar dislocation or subtalar dislocation may also mimic an ankle fracture. Infection and Charcot arthropathy can be differentiated by the results of history and physical examination, although radiographs make the diagnosis.

Etiology or pathophysiology

Caused by a twisting injury. The most common classification system, Lauge-Hansen, is based on the "twisting" sequence and is divided into four categories of ankle fractures: supination-external rotation (SER), pronation-external rotation (PER), supination-adduction (SA), and pronation-abduction (PA). Each category is further subdivided into stages of increasing severity: SER I to IV, PER I to IV, SA I and II, and PA I to III. The Weber classification is based on the level of fibular fracture in relation to the syndesmosis on the medial side. A Weber A fracture is a fibula fracture below the syndesmosis; Weber B is at or near the syndesmosis; and Weber C is above the syndesmosis and indicates a syndesmotic disruption. Assessment of the syndesmosis becomes crucial in the evaluation of ankle fractures.

Epidemiology

Ankle fractures are the most common type of fracture seen by orthopedic surgeons. The SER type comprises about 50% to 75% of all ankle fractures. The other three types each account for approximately 5% to 10%. Ankle fractures are becoming more prevalent, especially in patients who sustain trauma, as improved restraint devices help accident victims survive.

Treatment

Nonsurgical
Nonsurgical treatment of ankle fractures is isolated to fractures that involve only one side (usually lateral). Small tip avulsions of either side can also be treated in a cast. The most common fracture pattern seen for nonsurgical treatment is an SER II.

Surgical
The bimalleolar or trimalleolar fracture and its equivalent injuries require open reduction and internal fixation because of the highly unstable patterns present in these fractures. Reduction and fixation are usually accomplished with plating of the lateral side and screw fixation of the medial side. If the medial-sided injury is ligamentous in nature, there is no need to open the medial side unless the deltoid has flipped into the joint and is preventing reduction. The posterior malleolus fracture usually reduces with fixation of the fibula, which obviates the need for fixation. If it does not reduce or if the fragment is extremely large (usually greater than 25% of the articular surface), fixation is usually warranted. This can be done with screw fixation from either an anterior to posterior direction or the reverse. The ankle syndesmosis should always be stressed after fixation to assess for disruption and the need for a syndesmosis screw. The screw may be three or four cortices and may or may not require removal. This controversial decision is entirely surgeon's preference.

Exercise and activity modification
Patients who are prone to ankle sprains may use some ankle support or high-top shoes during sporting activities to help prevent recurrent injuries; some of these aids may ultimately lead to a fracture. Exercise and activity modification is inherent to the treatment plan, whether surgical or nonsurgical. All usually require non–weight-bearing for 6 to 8 weeks. After the fracture is healed, aggressive rehabilitation of motion, proprioception, and strength of the ankle is necessary. Rehabilitate with a home exercise program.

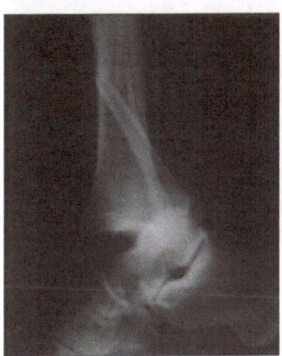

Figure 1. Lateral radiograph of an ankle fracture dislocation of the right ankle.

Treatment aims
Surgical: To restore the normal anatomy of the ankle mortise, to provide rigid fixation to prevent redisplacement, and to allow early motion.
Nonsurgical: To provide adequate immobilization to allow the fracture to heal in acceptable alignment.

Prognosis
Overall, the prognosis is excellent. With nonsurgical treatment, SER II fractures have healing rates of 98%. The rate of good to excellent results in ankle fractures at 3 years or more is 85% to 90%. Long-term morbidity is usually associated with chronic swelling, which can last up to a year, or with hardware pain necessitating removal.

Follow-up and management
Surgical: Depending on the patient's reliability, early motion out of a cast can be instituted after the initial splint postoperatively. Non–weight-bearing should be maintained for 6 weeks; some physicians, however, allow immediate weight bearing (with or without a cast or Cam Walker), with similar results and no loss of fixation. Postoperative therapy should be instituted to strengthen the ankle and calf and restore motion and proprioception.
Nonsurgical: To prevent weight bearing, patients usually wear a cast for 6 weeks or until the fracture is radiographically or clinically healed. Some physicians have instituted early weight bearing in this group as well. The same physical therapy is prescribed.

Key references
1. Geisler WB, Tsao AK, Hughes JL: Fractures and injuries of the ankle. In *Rockwood and Green's Fractures in Adults* edn 4. Edited by Rockwood CA, Green DP, Bucholz RW, et al. Philadelphia: Lippincott Williams and Wilkins; 1996:2201–2266.
2. Griend RV, Michelson JD, Bone LB: Fractures of the ankle and the distal part of the tibia. In *Instructional Course Lectures.* Edited by Springfield DS. Rosemont, IL: American Academy of Orthopaedic Surgeons; 1997, 46:311–321.
3. Michelson JD: Fractures about the ankle. *J Bone Joint Surg* 1995, 77A:142–152.

Diagnosis

History

Anterior cruciate ligament (ACL) tears usually occur in athletically active people in their second and third decades of life. There is usually no prodromal history of pain or swelling. The injury typically occurs in one of three mechanisms of injury: deceleration with knee valgus and leg external rotation, knee hyperextension and internal rotation, or a direct blow to the knee producing an exaggerated hyperextension or valgus motion to the knee. Frequently, an audible "pop" is heard and immediate swelling is noted. According to longitudinal studies, a "pop" and swelling are associated with at least a 75% incidence of a torn ACL. The athlete usually cannot continue playing at the time of injury. Recent studies have shown an increase of ACL ruptures in female athletes compared with male athletes in same sports (eg, high school and college basketball, soccer).

Physical findings

Immediately after injury, minimal swelling and pain may occur (within 2 hours of injury). On palpation, lateral joint tenderness is frequently present in the area of the midlateral one-third joint capsule (correlate to the anatomic area of a Segond's fracture). Patients often limp while attempting to walk and have incomplete active extension and flexion of the knee. The Lachman test is the most sensitive for an ACL rupture and is performed with the knee partially flexed (25°), the femur stabilized with one hand, and the tibia pulled forward with the other (Fig. 1). The examiner feels for translation (distance traveled) of the tibia on the femur and for the end point (how abruptly the tibia stops) of translation. Increased translation and a soft or "boggy" end point are objective findings of an ACL tear. The contralateral normal knee is used for comparison. False-negative examinations often occur secondary to pain and hamstring musculature spasm. Use of the stabilized Lachman test (examiner's thigh under the injured knee) can aid in examination and improve patient comfort and relaxation (Fig. 2). The pivot shift is a dynamic test that passively flexes or extends the knee producing tibiofemoral subluxation to reproduce knee joint instability. The result is positive for an ACL tear when an abrupt shift of the tibia on the femur is noted.

Imaging and laboratory studies

Radiographs are usually normal. An avulsion fracture of the lateral tibial cortex is the sine qua non of a cruciate ligament tear (ACL or posterior cruciate ligament) and is termed a *Segond's fracture*. Magnetic resonance imaging is very sensitive for diagnosis of ACL ruptures and for concomitant tears of collateral ligaments, menisci, and osteochondral impaction injuries (bone bruises). Osteochondral injuries are common (80% in acute ACL tears) and occur most frequently on the posterior aspect of the lateral tibial condyle and the anterior aspect of the lateral femoral condyle. An effusion on T2-weighted images is also common (Fig. 3).

Complications

Failure to diagnose an ACL tear is common because the patient usually quickly regains the ability to walk once the acute pain and swelling resolve. Injury to the knee usually recurs if the patient continues to engage in jumping-, cutting-, and twisting-type activities after injury. Arthritis can be considered a complication of the natural history or the surgical treatment of ACL and meniscal tears.

Differential diagnosis
A patellar dislocation with spontaneous reduction frequently mimics an ACL tear (ie, an audible pop, swelling, and visual subluxation can occur). In such a patellar injury, the result of a Lachman test is negative and tenderness is noted in the medial aspect of the superior patella.

Etiology or pathophysiology
Recent information confirms the increased incidence of ACL impairment in females in noncontact injuries. Hypotheses include poor jump training, anatomic differences such as genu valgum, a wider pelvis, and a narrowed intercondylar femoral notch.

Epidemiology
Recent longitudinal studies have defined ACL injury rates with an emphasis on male versus female rates. Increased rates of noncontact injuries occur in females in basketball, soccer, and football in high school and in college.

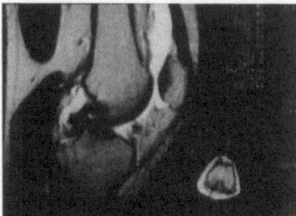

Figure 1. Magnetic resonance image of torn ACL fibers.

Treatment

Nonsurgical

Initial treatment involves short-term management of pain and swelling and return of normal range of motion and a functional gait pattern. The thigh musculature should be strengthened or at least maintained. Nonsurgical management involves bracing of the affected knee during activities that present a risk for ACL tears. Bracing fails in one third to two thirds of patients, depending on the population studied. Nonsurgical treatment is usually recommended for patients with lower activity demands and those with preexisting arthritis.

Surgical

Indications for surgical repair usually involve the continued desire to perform activities that present a risk for ACL tears. Surgical repair of the torn ends has routinely failed. Reconstruction or replacement of the torn ligament ends is recommended with autograft of the mid-one-third patellar tendon or autograft hamstring for primary ACL reconstruction; allograft of the patellar or Achilles tendon is used less often than autograft. Arthroscopically assisted techniques are used to minimize incisions and treat associated meniscal or osteochondral injuries. After surgery, range of motion of the knee is required to prevent stiffness.

Exercise and activity modification

Prevention of ACL injuries is controversial. Numerous studies have provided arguments for and against use of bracing during football. Bracing is often used for linemen and linebackers. Jumping and flexibility training has recently been used in female athletes to decrease ACL injuries. Nonsurgical management of ACL tears requires avoidance of cutting-, twisting-, jumping-type sporting injuries. Straight-ahead jogging and bicycling are usually well tolerated by an athlete with an ACL-deficient knee.

Treatment aims
To provide a stable knee with full range of motion and strength.

Prognosis
Excellent if proper technique and postoperative rehabilitation (in the clinic and at home) are instituted. Full range of motion obtained before surgery is important for full recovery.

Follow-up and management
Immediate range-of-motion exercises and weight bearing after surgical reconstruction of the torn ACL are useful physical therapy techniques. Concomitant injures (meniscal tears, osteochondral fractures) affect timing of weight bearing and range of motion after surgery. Return to sports is controversial and usually involves 4 to 6 months of healing and rehabilitation. Bracing after surgery is controversial but is usually unnecessary 1 year after reconstruction.

Key references

1. Johnson DL, Urban WP Jr, Caborn DNM, et al.: Articular cartilage changes seen with magnetic resonance imaging-detected bone bruises associated with anterior cruciate ligament rupture. Am J Sports Med 1998, 26:409-414.

2. Schenck RC, Lance ED, Holmes CF, et al.: A prospective outcome study of home rehabilitation programs following ACL reconstructions. Arthroscopy 1997, 13:285-290.

3. Shelbourne KD, Wilckens JH, Mollabasky A: Arthrofibrosis in acute ACL reconstruction: the effect of timing of reconstruction and rehabilitation. Am J Sports Med 1991, 19:332-336.

4. Daniel DM, Stone ML, Dobson BE, et al.: Fate of the ACL injured patient: a prospective outcome study. Am J Sports Med 1994, 22:632-644.

Diagnosis

History
Careful history and physical examination are the most important factors in diagnosing glenohumeral dislocation.

Define mechanism of injury: position of arm, amount of applied force, point of force application.

Injury occurs with arm in extended, abducted, and externally rotated position.

Important to document amount of trauma that initiated instability and force required to produce subsequent episodes.

History of shoulder dislocation and previous treatment.

Physical findings
Extreme pain.

Muscle spasm.

Humeral head palpable anteriorly.

Posterior sulcus sign: hollow beneath the acromion posteriorly.

Arm held in slight abduction and external rotation.

Patient incapable of complete internal rotation and abduction.

Important to document radial, median, ulnar, musculocutaneous, and axillary nerve function before and after reduction (axillary nerve injury is associated with anterior dislocation).

Imaging and laboratory studies
Need to document: direction of dislocation, associated fractures, and barriers to relocation.

Radiographs: anteroposterior, axillary lateral/scapula Y views.

Axillary lateral: often shows head compression, glenoid, or lesser tuberosity fractures.

Scapula Y view: cassette is placed anteriorly lateral to the deltoid; scapula is positioned perpendicular to the cassette, beam is placed parallel to the spine of the scapula, scapula projects as a Y.

Anterior dislocation: humeral head anterior to Y.

Three orthogonal projections of the shoulder.

If at least two views 90° to one another cannot be obtained, computed tomography or magnetic resonance imaging may be helpful.

Hill-Sachs lesion: defect on posterolateral aspect of humeral head (where head rests against glenoid).

Bankart lesion: bony fragment involved is noted on anterior-inferior aspect of glenoid.

Complications
Avulsion of the anterior-inferior glenohumeral ligament and capsule.

Fracture of the glenoid, humeral head, and tuberosities.

Rotator cuff tears: frequency increases with age; after age 60 years, 80% incidence.

Vascular injuries: more common in elderly patients; axillary artery or vein, respective branches.

Nerve injuries: axillary nerve most commonly injured.

Recurrent instability.

Differential diagnosis
If the patient has an acute anterior dislocation, it is difficult to suspect anything else.
Important to diagnose anterior, inferior, or posterior dislocation.
Evaluation for other associated injuries, including fractures.

Etiology or pathophysiology
Traumatic
Shoulder abduction, extension, and external rotation.
Chronic instability.
Voluntary dislocation.

Epidemiology
45% of all dislocations involve the glenohumeral joint.
Anterior dislocations account for 85% of glenohumeral dislocations.
Subcoracoid is the most common anterior dislocation.

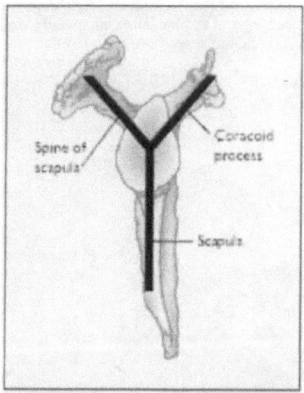

Spine of scapula

Coracoid process

Scapula

Figure 1. Anatomic scapula Y view.

Treatment

Nonsurgical

Important to reduce the dislocation as soon as possible; it is helpful to obtain complete radiographs before reduction to rule out fractures.

Early relocation reduces neurovascular compromise, decreases muscle spasm, decreases chance of increase in size of Hill-Sachs lesion.

Intravenous sedation is often required to provide adequate relaxation for reduction. Intra-articular lidocaine (20 mL of 1% plain lidocaine) is an alternative to intravenous sedation.

Reduction is obtained using traction and countertraction.

Obtain postreduction radiograph to verify reduction.

Postreduction physical examination should verify neurovascular status—radial, median, ulnar, musculocutaneous, and axillary nerves; radial and ulnar pulses.

Surgical

If attempts at closed reduction fail, open reduction may be necessary.

Soft tissue interposition (subscapularis, biceps) can prevent closed reduction.

Axillary artery, axillary nerve, and brachial plexus can be in altered anatomic position secondary to the dislocation.

Deltopectoral approach.

External rotation and lateral traction disimpact the humeral head from the glenoid.

Gentle reduction of head into glenoid visualizing articular surface.

Displaced greater tuberosity fracture.

For glenoid rim fracture, surgery is indicated if intra-articular incongruity or inadequate glenoid arc exists.

Exercise and activity modification

Activity modification may be important in the patient with recurrent dislocations. If activity modification is not an option, surgical reconstruction may be necessary.

Treatment aims
To reduce dislocation, document associated injuries (fractures, neurovascular), and prevent recurrence.

Prognosis
Recurrence rates are 55% to 90%.

Follow-up and management
Optimize shoulder stability
Protection, muscle rehabilitation.
Sling for 1 to 2 weeks. Range of motion: at least 90° forward flexion, 0° external rotation at 3 weeks. Deltoid/cuff isometrics.
Range of motion of elbow. Begin rotator cuff strengthening program at 3 weeks; swimming at 6 weeks.
Resume sports/overhead activities with normal rotator cuff strength, full forward elevation, and no apprehension.

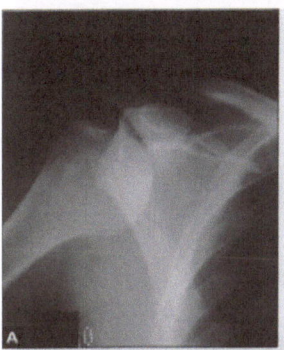 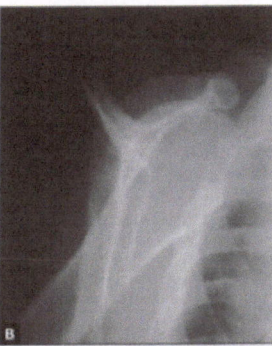

Figure 2. A, Anteroposterior view with anterior dislocation. B, Scapula Y view with anterior dislocation.

Key references
1. Matsen FA III, Thomas SC, Rockwood CA, et al: Glenohumeral instability. In *The Shoulder* edn 2, vol 2. Edited by Rockwood CA Jr, Matsen FA III. Philadelphia: WB Saunders; 1998:611–741.
2. Pollock RG, Bigliani LU: Glenohumeral instability: evaluation and treatment. *J Am Assoc Orthop Surg* 1993, 1:24–32.

Diagnosis

History

Significant back pain alters a child's lifestyle, and pain at night is especially serious. Back pain that is associated with mild trauma and is improving tends to resolve spontaneously in weeks, but worsening back pain without clear cause deserves aggressive work-up. Pain radiating from the back into the buttocks is probably due to localized musculoskeletal strain, but pain radiating into the lower extremities may be due to disk herniation or other mass lesions of the spine. Symptoms such as muscle weakness, dysuria, or frank urinary or fecal incontinence associated with back pain suggest a serious spinal neurologic lesion. Adolescents tend to have either mechanical back pain, such as that seen in adults, or, infrequently, a herniated disk. Significant back pain in younger children, especially those 10 years of age or younger, may be due to extremely serious spinal disease, which requires detailed work-up.

Physical Findings

Back examination reveals localized tenderness of the paravertebral muscles, muscle spasm that does not relax with marching in place, limited forward flexion of the spine, lateral shift of the spine away from the painful side, and, at times, scoliosis. On examination of the extremities, buttock/thigh ache occurring on a straight-leg raise suggests mechanical back pain; severe pain radiating down the extremity (sciatica) with the same maneuver represents a positive result on a straight-leg test and suggests a herniated disk. Both lower and upper extremities are tested for muscle strength, deep tendon reflexes, and skin sensation. Isolated muscle atrophy strongly suggests a nerve root lesion.

Imaging and laboratory studies

Radiographs: for initial screening, a standing anteroposterior and lateral radiograph of the entire spine is obtained. If scoliosis is present, the degree and location are assessed. Curves without vertebral rotation are usually "functional" and are due to muscle spasm only; those with rotation or other vertebral structural changes suggest a primary spine disease process.

Special studies: subtle bony lesions can be detected by bone scanning; computed tomography can be used to define congenital lesions; and herniated disk, osteomyelitis, and spinal cord tumor are best studied with magnetic resonance imaging.

Laboratory tests: complete blood count with erythrocyte sedimentation rate; measurement of C-reactive protein level; blood cultures for infection; and measurement of calcium, phosphate, alkaline phosphatase, and uric acid levels for tumor work-up.

Complications

The complications of back pain depend on the cause. Mechanical back pain seldom has complications. Herniated disk may cause muscle weakness, such as that seen with foot drop. Fracture, if severe, may cause neurologic injury. Progressive spondylolisthesis is associated with lumbar "swayback," and neurologic lesions may develop. Untreated infection and vertebral or spinal cord tumor can result in spinal instability and paralysis.

Differential diagnosis
Pyelonephitis.
Pneumonia.
Soft tissue abscess.

Etiology
Mechanical back pain, muscle strain, contusion.
Herniated disk.
Osteomyelitis.
Eosinophilic granuloma.
Scheuermann's disease.
Spondylolisthesis or spondylolysis.
Vertebral tumor: osteoblastoma.
Diastematomyelia.
Fracture: wedge, compression, or burst.
Dysraphism: myelomeningocele, congenital scoliosis, dural ectasia diskitis.
Osteoid osteoma.
Spinal cord tumor.
Ankylosing spondylitis.

Epidemiology
Whereas 60% to 80% of adults have intermittent back pain of mechanical origin, back pain in children is extremely rare. In many children with back pain lasting more than a few days, the pain has an underlying musculoskeletal or neurologic cause.

Treatment

Nonsurgical
For mechanical back pain, nonsteroidal anti-inflammatory drugs are used for 4 weeks. This therapy is contraindicated in patients with gastrointestinal disorders, especially ulcers. The main side effect is gastrointestinal distress. Back and abdominal exercises can help relieve symptoms in patients with mechanical back pain. For patients with Scheuermann's disease, temporary back bracing may be needed.

Surgical
In children with mechanical back pain, surgery is not indicated. For herniated disks, failure of conservative treatment may require diskectomy. Progressive spondylolisthesis or painful spondylolysis may require fusion. Osteomyelitis requires long-term antibiotic therapy and possibly biopsy or debridement. A tumor almost always requires surgery.

Exercise and activity modification
A healthy, active lifestyle that maintains ideal body weight probably reduces the risk for common mechanical back pain in children. Patients with severe active back pain are placed on bed rest for 1 week; physical education and athletic activities are restricted until symptoms resolve. Most cases of back pain in children resolve with this temporary reduction in activities.

Treatment aims
To relieve the symptoms of back pain and allow the child to return to normal activities.

Prognosis
Most mechanical back pain resolves in several weeks after activity levels have been reduced. Pain due to a herniated disk can resolve with 1 to 2 weeks of bed rest and 1 to 3 months of avoidance of sports. Spondylolisthesis or spondylolysis symptoms may begin to lessen with 2 to 4 weeks of activity reduction. In most patients, Scheuermann's disease also responds to activity reduction within weeks. The prognosis of patients with tumor, infection, and congenital anomalies is based on the severity of disease at time of diagnosis.

Follow-up and management
Frequent follow-up (weekly) is needed during the initial phases of severe back pain. If tumor, infection, or other severe spinal disease is suspected, rapid work-up is indicated. Follow-up is needed until all symptoms have resolved.

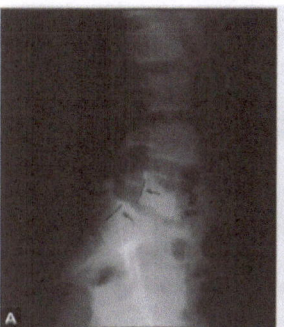 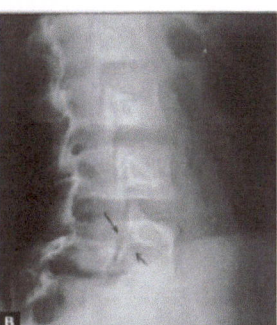

Figure 1. A, Low back pain caused by spondylolysis of L5-S1 in a patient aged 17 years. Note lucency in the pars interarticularis. B, A lateral radiograph showing Grade II spondylolisthesis with forward displacement of L5 on S1.

Key references
1. Hensinger RH: Current concepts review: spondylolysis and spondylolisthesis in children and adolescents. *J Bone Joint Surg [Am]* 1989, 71:1098.

R.C. Schenck, Jr.

Diagnosis

History
Patients with a Baker's cyst present with intermittent posterior knee and proximal calf pain. The patient usually notes swelling or a palpable mass or cyst that changes in size with activity level. Pain and swelling are usually related to walking or standing activities.

Physical findings
A palpable mass is usually seen in the posteromedial aspect of the knee. Acute tenderness is rare, but aching and pain occur on deep palpation. Concomitant knee abnormality is common and can be caused by many conditions, including arthritis, meniscal tears, or related effusions.

Imaging and laboratory studies
Plain radiographs usually reveal mild to moderate arthritis. Magnetic resonance imaging is diagnostic and shows cystic formation ("hernia") between the medial head of the gastrocnemius and pes anserine tendons. The cyst can be of multiple shapes and sizes and, because it is filled with fluid, will have a high signal on T2-weighted images (Fig. 1).

Complications
There are no special complications.

Differential diagnosis
Because of its mass effect, a Baker's cyst can mimic a posterior knee tumor. A Baker's cyst can rupture, resulting in calf swelling and pain that mimic deep venous thrombosis of the calf venous system. Such a presentation is denoted pseudo-thrombophlebitis syndrome.

Etiology or pathophysiology
A Baker's cyst is most commonly the result of intra-articular knee abnormality, with the resultant joint effusion and pressure producing a cystic hernia of joint capsule between the medial head of the gastrocnemius and pes anserinus tendons.

Epidemiology
Baker's cyst can occur at any age but is most common in middle-aged or older adults.

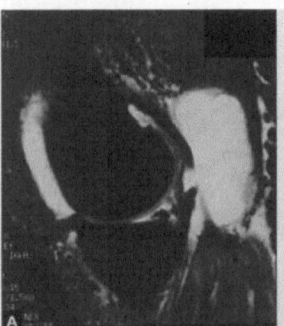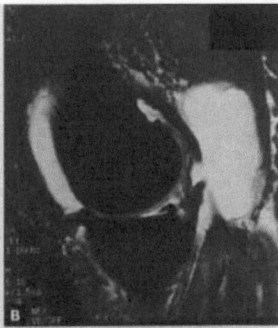

Figure 1. Transverse, T2-weighted magnetic resonance image of a typical Baker's cyst. A and B, Note the differences in the size and shape of the cyst.

Treatment

Nonsurgical

Baker's cysts are always treated nonsurgically first, with therapy directed toward the intra-articular abnormality. Nonsteroidal anti-inflammatory drugs (NSAIDs) are usually given first. COX-2 inhibitors, new lines of NSAIDs, are also useful. Bracing may help decrease arthritis symptoms and thus, in time, decrease the symptoms associated with a Baker's cyst. Injection of the knee with a corticosteroid preparation (*ie*, Celestone; Schering, Kenilworth, NJ) can alleviate the intra-articular abnormality when NSAIDs have failed. As a general rule, only three such injections should be given per year. Aspiration of a large cyst with injections of a corticosteroid can reduce the size of the cyst and hasten resolution.

Surgical

Surgical treatment is focused on the intra-articular abnormality. Treatment usually involves management of meniscal tear or arthritis. Arthroscopic treatment of the intra-articular knee abnormality with simultaneous aspiration and injection (corticosteroids) of the Baker's cyst is a common approach. Exploration and excision of a loculated symptomatic cyst is rarely necessary. In contrast, resection/exploration of a Baker's cyst is done rarely; this procedure is generally not recommended because it is associated with a high recurrence rate. Frequently, the recurrent cyst is larger than the original because of the enlarged hernia created to allow resection. The patient should be counseled on these aspects of a Baker's cyst and the chronicity of the condition when considering treatment options.

Exercise and activity modification

A generalized rehabilitation program of the thigh musculature usually helps alleviate knee symptoms and related bursal swelling.

Treatment aims

To decrease symptoms related to intra-articular knee abnormality and posterior knee swelling and pain.

Prognosis

Improvement in symptoms is good. Complete elimination of a Baker's cyst is difficult but rarely requires surgical excision. The risk for recurrence accompanies surgical excision.

Follow-up and management

Recovery after surgical treatment involves rehabilitation of the specific knee procedure (eg, arthroscopic debridement, total knee replacement). Recurrence of the cyst and progression of knee degeneration should be anticipated.

Key references

1. Childress HM: Posterior medial meniscal lesions and popliteal cysts. *J Bone Joint Surg* 1965, 47A:1272.

2. Kattamis AC, Gomez J, Schenck RC: Pseudothrombophlebitis (PTP) syndrome in an adolescent without rheumatic disease: a case report. *Clin Orthop Rel Res* 1994, 308:250–253.

Diagnosis

History

Rupture of the long head tendon of the biceps usually occurs in middle-aged or older patients with chronic bicipital tendonitis secondary to an impingement syndrome or rotator cuff tear. Patients may have a history of repetitive use of the arm in overhead activity. Pain is less intense at rest and worsens with use. Avulsion of the biceps tendon at the elbow is rare and usually occurs during a heavy lift. Unlike proximal injuries, preinjury symptoms are uncommon.

Physical findings

Proximal injuries demonstrate tenderness in the bicipital groove. The area of maximal tenderness should change with rotation of the arm and may disappear with internal rotation as the biceps tendon moves under the conjoined tendons. Ecchymosis in the arm is seen occasionally with acute ruptures. For distal ruptures, moderate to severe pain occurs in the antecubital fossa and is associated with tenderness, swelling, and ecchymosis. Distal deformity, weakness, and a palpable defect are usually present, but elbow flexion is preserved because of an intact brachialis.

Imaging and laboratory findings

Routine radiographs of the shoulder and arm are usually normal. Although the use of ultrasonography to evaluate the biceps has become popular, the imaging study of choice is magnetic resonance imaging (MRI). MRI can show the normal biceps musculotendinous relationships and can accurately reveal associated lesions such as a rotator cuff tear.

Complications

The most common complication of a proximal biceps tendon rupture is failure to recognize an associated rotator cuff tear. Most of these tears occur in older patients and can be treated expectantly. However, if the patient is young (55 years of age or younger), surgical repair provides a strong shoulder for overhead work and sports. Biceps rupture has also been associated with proximal humerus fracture and dislocations and injury to the brachial plexus. Although only slight loss of function occurs with proximal ruptures of the biceps, rupture of the distal biceps predictably causes significant loss of flexion and supination strengths.

Differential diagnosis

Impingement syndrome.
Rheumatoid arthritis or osteoarthritis.
Glenohumeral instability.
Glenoid labral tear.

Etiology or pathophysiology

The cause is usually multifactorial. Chief among proximal ruptures is the anatomic location of the tendon where it is involved in impingement between the acromion and the humeral head. In distal ruptures, injury usually occurs during a heavy load with the elbow flexed 90°. Rupture results with sudden or prolonged contraction of the muscle against high load resistance.

Epidemiology

The incidence of frank ruptures of the biceps tendon is 5%. The most common age group at the time of injury is between 45 and 55 years of age. Bilateral involvement is noted in 8% of cases.

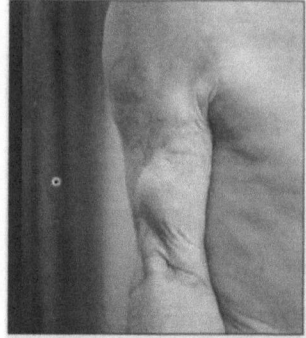

Figure 1. A male patient aged 67 years with a chronic rupture of the long head tendon of the biceps.

Treatment

Nonsurgical

Most ruptures of the proximal biceps tendon are associated with rotator cuff tears and can be treated expectantly. Initially, the patient should avoid painful activities and is told to rest the extremity, apply ice followed by moist heat, and perform simple range-of-motion exercises. As symptoms improve, rehabilitation exercises (warm-up, stretching, and strengthening exercises for the rotator cuff, deltoid, and elbow flexors) are instituted. Distal injuries of the biceps tendon should be managed surgically.

Surgical

Younger, active patients with proximal ruptures of the biceps and most patients with distal ruptures of the biceps are managed surgically. Although functional loss is minimal with proximal injury (if the short head tendon of the biceps is intact at its coracoid origin), rupture of the distal biceps results in significant loss of flexion and supination strength. Thus, treatment of acute ruptures involves surgical repair, whereas chronic injuries are usually addressed by repairing the tendon to the brachialis tendon or the coronoid process of the ulna.

Exercise and activity modification

See Nonsurgical Treatment section.

Treatment aims
Return of strength and function.

Prognosis
Prognosis is excellent for nearly full return of strength and function with proximal injuries.
Weakness and pain with resisted elbow flexion are noted with nonoperative management of distal injuries.
Return to work and sports after motion and strength have returned to within 90% of normal.

Follow-up and management (or rehabilitation)
Posterior elbow splint for 7 to 10 days. Range-of-motion exercises without resistance for 4 to 6 weeks. Progressive increase in activities after 6 weeks.

Key references
1. Burkhead WZ: The biceps tendon. In The Shoulder, vol 2. Edited by Rockwood CA Jr, Matsen FA III. Philadelphia: W.B. Saunders; 1998:1009–1063.
2. Morrey BF, Askew LJ, An KN, et al.: Rupture of the distal tendon of the biceps brachii: a biomechanical study. J Bone Joint Surg [Am] 1985, 67:418–421.

Diagnosis

History

Bipartite patella is usually asymptomatic and is an anomalous or radiographic finding. Symptoms related to the detached portion of the patella are anterior knee pain and frequent lateral-sided patellofemoral pain. Patients usually have no history of injury. As with any patellofemoral condition, symptoms associated with descending stairs (eg, pain) are usually greater than those associated with climbing stairs (the center of gravity is further away as one descends stairs; thus, the fulcrum is longer and the knee more painful in contrast to climbing stairs, where the center of gravity is closer to the knee axis secondary to leaning forward).

Physical findings

Bipartite patella is laterally located on the patella and can usually be palpated as an enlargement on the superior and lateral aspect. Range of motion is usually full, and ligamentous examination yields normal findings. Patellar tenderness, when present, is usually lateral and involves the bipartite portion of the patella.

Imaging and laboratory studies

Plain radiographs are usually diagnostic and should include a tangential view of the patellofemoral joint (eg, a Merchant's or "sunrise" view). Magnetic resonance imaging is also diagnostic but should be ordered specifically for evaluation of the patella. This test is also useful for ruling out meniscal and other conditions. Plain radiographs of the contralateral knee should be obtained to rule out bilateral involvement. Presence of a marginal fracture of the patella can be difficult to detect on radiographs alone and requires physical examination.

Complications

Bipartite patella can be an asymptomatic condition associated with another abnormality. Treatment should not be based on radiographic findings alone (Fig. 1).

Differential diagnosis
Any developmental condition can be bilateral and should be suspected. Treatment should focus on concomitant patellofemoral symptoms rather than on the bony abnormality. Tripartite patella and patellar fracture ("marginal" fracture) should be suspected when radiography shows multiple ossification sites and sharp fracture edges, respectively.

Etiology or pathophysiology
The development of the patella and incomplete fusion of the anomalous ossification centers causes the sesamoid (patella) to be in two separate but firmly connected parts.

Epidemiology
Bipartite patella occurs in 1% to 2% of the general population and, because it is an anomalous condition, is usually asymptomatic.

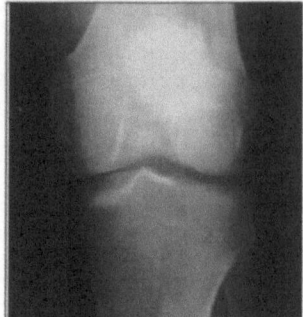

Figure 1. Radiograph of a bipartite patella.

20

Treatment

Nonsurgical

Management of patellar symptoms is usually the most common avenue of treatment. Quadriceps stretching, hamstring stretching, patellar taping (eg, McConnell taping), and patellofemoral bracing are standard.

Surgical

Surgical treatment should be limited to symptomatic patients in whom conservative or nonoperative treatment fails. Treatment usually involves arthroscopy, removal of any loose or detached fragments, and reattachment of the quadriceps tendon. Excision of a large fragment should be performed rarely with excision because doing so may cause pain from the limited remaining patellar articular surface. A lateral release is indicated for pain, but only in patients who did not respond to conservative treatment.

Exercise and activity modification

See Nonsurgical Treatment section.

Treatment aims
To relieve pain and increase function.

Prognosis
Bipartite patella usually becomes symptomatic in the second or third decade of life and is associated with overuse. Conservative management of patellofemoral symptoms should be continued for several months before surgery is performed. Conservative management is successful in approximately 70% to 80% of cases. Surgical management is also successful if combined with initial nonoperative management.

Follow-up and management
Continued follow-up of conservative management, documenting an increase in quadriceps strength, is necessary to ensure patient compliance. Lateral release requires that range of motion be ensured. In addition, patients should be informed that lateral swelling will be present for several months after a lateral retinacular release.

Key references
1. Adams JD, Leonard RD: Developmental anomaly of the patella frequently diagnosed as a fracture. *Surg Gynecol Obstet* 1925, 41:601–604.
2. Carter SR: Traumatic separation of a bipartite patella. *Imaging* 1989, 20:244.

Diagnosis

History

Contact with animals or altercations with humans.

Patient may deny being in a fight because of embarrassment (Fig. 1).

Physical findings

Pain.

Fever.

Swelling.

Decreased motion at affected joint, usually the metaphalangeal or distal interphalangeal.

Erythema.

Swelling.

Swollen nodes and, often, infection; systemic signs of fever, leukocytosis.

With any laceration over the metaphalangeal or proximal interphalangeal joint, a human bite wound must be strongly suspected.

Imaging and laboratory studies

Radiography

Complete blood count to determine presence of leukocytosis

For animal bite, status of animal's vaccination records.

Patient's tetanus immunization status.

Differential diagnosis

Anything that can produce a wound: sharp objects, thorn, splinter. Careful history if any suspicion of a human bite.

Bite from insect, particularly brown recluse spider.

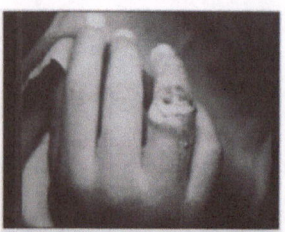

Figure 1. Neglected human bite infections, secondary to street fighting, often involve the proximal interpha-langeal joints of the digits as well as the metaphalangeal joints. Because of the organisms involved and the possibility of septic arthritis, these are serious problems that should be treated with surgical decompression and appropriate antibiotics. They are often neglected because the patient might not present the appropriate history or because the physician overlooks the fact that the wound may have been caused by a human bite.

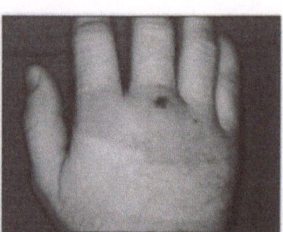

Figure 2. The cat bite illustrated on this hand appears innocuous because of the small puncture wound involved. However, such bites can develop into a severe problem because of the organisms harbored in the cat's mouth. Any suspected animal or human bite around a joint should be treated as an open joint and as a significant cause of hand impairment.

Treatment

Nonsurgical
The hand should be splinted and elevated, and the patient should be prescribed broad-spectrum antibiotics until cultures with specific organisms are available. Particular attention should be given to the organism *Eikenella corrodens* in human bites and to *Pasteurella multocida* in animal bites.

Tetanus prophylaxis.

Rabies immunization if indicated.

Surgical
Suppurative infection of any joint requires surgery.

Exercise and activity modification
No apparent relationship.

Treatment aims
To eradicate infection and preserve function.

Prognosis
Usually good if the bite is caught early. Cat bites are often more difficult to treat than human bites (Fig. 2).

Key references
1. Arons MS, Fernando L, Polayes IM: *Pasturella multicida:* the major cause of hand infections following domestic animal bites. *J Hand Surg* 1982, 7:47–52.
2. Farmer CB, Mann RJ: Human bite infections of the hand. *South Med J* 1966, 59:515–518.
3. Goldstein EJC, Barones MF, Miller TA: *Eikenella corrodens* in hand infections. *J Hand Surg* 1983, 8:563–567.
4. Mann RJ, Hoffeld TA, Farmer CB: Human bites of the hand: twenty years' experience. *J Hand Surg* 1977, 2:97–104.

Diagnosis

History

Most often associated with trauma to the to the proximal interphalangeal joint of the finger with progressive flexion contracture (Fig. 1).

Physical findings

Pain over the dorsum of the proximal interphalangeal (PIP) joint.

Inability to extend fully the PIP joint.

Swelling around the PIP joint.

In established boutonniere deformities, there will be a flexion contracture of the PIP joint with an extension contractive of the distal interphalangeal joint.

In established contractures, there is always decreased range of motion in both proximal and distal interphalangeal joints.

Imaging and laboratory studies

Radiography may show an avulsed bony fragment off the middle phalanx, if the central slip is avulsed from the middle phalanx with a small fracture.

Complications

Permanent contracture of distal interphalangeal (DIP) joint (Fig. 2).

Permanent loss of motion.

Skin over PIP joint may become attenuated.

Differential diagnosis

Fracture or fracture-dislocation of the PIP joint.

Pseudoboutonniere deformity.

Infection.

Etiology or pathophysiology

Disruption of the central slip of the extensor apparatus that allows the lateral band to sublux volarly. Attenuation of the central slip in patients with rheumatoid arthritis or burns.

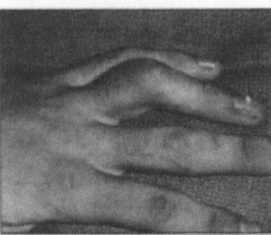

Figure 1. The cause of the boutonniere deformity is a tear of the central slip of the extensor mechanism. This tear allows the lateral bands to retract volarly to the axis of motion of the PIP joint, which results in a flexion contracture of the PIP joint and an extension contracture of the distal interphalangeal joint.

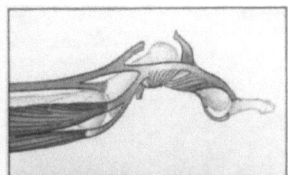

Figure 2. An untreated boutonniere deformity results in a fixed flexion contracture of the PIP joint and an extension contracture of the DIP joint, as shown in the ring finger of this patient's left hand.

Treatment

Nonsurgical
Pain relief may be provided by nonsteroidal anti-inflammatory drugs or analgesics.

Surgical
Initially, the treatment should be closed with splinting of the PIP joint in full extension for approximately 6 weeks. With the PIP joint splinted in extension, the DIP joint should be passively flexed several times during the day to keep the lateral bands from scarring.

Skin necrosis over the PIP joint is a complication of closed treatment.

An alternative to closed treatment is open repair of the central slip and possible pinning of the PIP joint in full extension with a Kirschner wire.

In chronic cases, a reconstruction of the central slip can be done using either tendon graft or available tissue at the site of the injury.

Exercise and activity modification
No special precautions necessary.

Treatment aims
To gain as much extension as possible in the PIP joint without limiting flexion.

Prognosis
Mild PIP-joint contractures can be tolerated without any treatment. Acute injuries that are treated with splinting usually do well. Surgical reconstruction usually leaves some residual deformity.

Follow-up and management
Any treatment, whether surgical or closed, needs passive flexion of the DIP joint to prevent lateral band scarring and extension contracture.

Key references

1. Nalebuff EA, Millender LH: Surgical treatment of the swan-neck deformity in rheumatoid arthritis. *Orthop Clin North Am* 1975, 6:733–753.
2. Rayan GM, Murray D: Classification and treatment of closed sagittal band injuries. *J Hand Surg* 1994, 19A:590–594.
3. Thompson JS, Littler JW, Upton J: The spiral oblique retinacular ligament (SORL). *J Hand Surg* 1978, 3:482–487.
4. Tonkin MA, Hughes J, Smith KL: Lateral band trans-location for swan-neck deformity. *J Hand Surg* 1992, 17A:260–267.
5. Urbaniak JR, Hayes MG: Chronic boutonniere deformity: an anatomic reconstruction. *J Hand Surg* 1981, 6:379–383.

Diagnosis

History
The chief symptoms of bunions are pain, redness, and swelling overlying the medial aspect of the first metatarsal head; they are associated with shoewear. Usually patients have no pain when they do not wear shoes; however, shoes that are too tight force the great toe into a valgus posture, exposing the metatarsal head to direct shoe pressure. The pain is aggravated by standing and walking and is relieved by getting off of one's feet and removing one's shoes.

Physical findings
When the patient stands, the great toe deviates laterally at the metatarsophalangeal joint, creating the hallux valgus deformity and making the first metatarsal head more prominent medially. The forefoot is frequently splayed. The great toe may deviate so far laterally that it overlaps or underlaps the second toe, creating deformity of this digit (Fig. 1). On palpation there is often tenderness over the prominent medial aspect of the first metatarsal head. Range of motion of the first metatarsophalangeal joint may be restricted, and this motion can be crepitant and painful. An associated flatfoot deformity is often noted.

Imaging and laboratory studies
Standing anteroposterior and lateral radiographs of the foot demonstrate the hallux valgus deformity, in which the angle between the shaft of the first metatarsal and the shaft of the proximal phalanx of the great toe is more than 20°. The base of the proximal phalanx is often shifted laterally, uncovering the first metatafsal head; on the medial aspect of the first metatarsal head, a bony prominence frequently develops. Arthritic changes are sometimes seen in the first metatarsophalangeal joint.

Differential diagnosis
Other conditions that can cause a painful first metatarsophalangeal joint of the great toe include gout and simple degenerative or posttraumatic arthritis of this joint. Neither of these conditions is associated with a severe hallux valgus deformity. Rheumatoid arthritis affecting the first metatarsophalangeal joint can also cause a hallux valgus deformity and a painful, prominent bunion.

Etiology or pathophysiology
Bunions occur more commonly in women, and development of this condition is associated with a definite genetic predisposition. The overriding cause of the deformity, however, is shoes that are too tight, particularly high-heeled, pointed-toed shoes. Wearing shoes of this shape for many years forces the toe into a fixed hallux valgus posture and exposes the first metatarsal head to irritation.

Epidemiology
Hallux valgus deformity may affect adolescents, particularly female adolescents, but the most commonly affected patients are women older than 50 years of age.

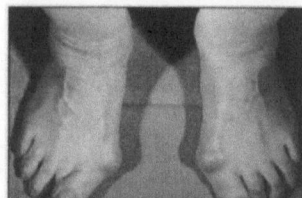

Figure 1. Photograph of a patient with bunions on both feet.

Treatment

Nonsurgical

Patients with symptomatic bunions should be advised carefully with regard to their shoewear. Most people wear shoes that are too small, and all patients with a symptomatic bunion should be prescribed an Oxford-type shoe with an extra-depth toe box that will allow sufficient room to accommodate the deformed toes. Donut-shaped pads can be applied over the bony prominences to relieve pressure. These pads should always be placed so that the pressure is relieved from the bony prominence and distributed around its periphery. If a patient has a flatfoot deformity, a simple longitudinal arch support can help to transfer the pressure of weight bearing off the forefoot and back into the arch of the foot. Night splints and exercise regimens have proven to be of little benefit in the nonoperative treatment of this problem. Activity modification should also be considered in the treatment of symptomatic bunions. Demanding activities, such as running and standing for prolonged periods, should be avoided and, obviously, judicious use of the proper shoewear should be of paramount importance.

Surgical

More than 100 different operations have been described to treat bunions and hallux valgus deformity. Many different factors come into play for the selection of the correct surgical treatment. Surgery should be reserved for those relatively rare patients whose symptoms have not been relieved through nonoperative means. The objectives of surgical treatment are to 1) remove the bunion prominence of the medial aspect of the first metatarsal head, 2) restore the alignment of the first ray to bring the first metatarsal parallel to the second metatarsal, and 3) to decrease the hallux valgus angle to less than 20°. These objectives can sometimes be accomplished with simple soft tissue releases and realignment; at other times, osteotomy, either at the base of the first metatarsal or through the head and neck of the first metatarsal, is necessary to restore the overall alignment of the first ray.

Exercise and activity modification

Improper shoewear contributes substantially to the creation of a hallux valgus deformity, and shoes that are too tight will rub against and irritate the prominent bunion. Strong efforts must sometimes be made to persuade patients to wear less cosmetically acceptable shoes that have a wide enough and deep enough toe box to accommodate their toes. Surgical treatment should never be offered for cosmesis alone; it should be limited to patients in whom nonsurgical treatment has failed and who have disabling forefoot pain.

Treatment aims

To relieve the pain over the bunion and to restore patients to a more productive and active lifestyle. Cosmesis should not be a consideration. Prophylactic surgery should not be recommended to prevent future problems.

Prognosis

Nonsurgical treatment often relieves the patient's symptoms sufficiently that no further treatment is necessary. When nonsurgical means fail, surgical correction followed by the use of appropriate shoewear can control symptoms for many years. Recovery from forefoot surgery is often prolonged, particularly when osteotomies are performed, and it may take as long as 6 months for patients to recover fully from bunion surgery.

Follow-up and management

After surgical correction, the foot must be protected from excessive weight bearing and toe motion for 6 to 8 weeks to allow healing of the osteotomies and soft tissue repair. Usually, this degree of protection and support can be accomplished with a wooden-soled postoperative shoe. After healing has occurred, vigorous active range-of-motion exercises for the toes and ankle should be undertaken to restore their function and minimize swelling. A gradually progressive walking program should be instituted to restore strength and mobility and to restore general physical fitness.

Key references

1. Coughlin MJ: Hallux valgus. *J Bone Joint Surg* 1996, 78:932–966.

2. Thompson FM, Coughlin MJ: The high price of high fashion footwear. *J Bone Joint Surg* 1994, 76A:1586–1593.

Diagnosis

History
Patients report painful swelling and redness over the lateral aspect of the fifth metatarsal head. The pain is aggravated by standing and walking, especially in tight shoewear. It is usually relieved by removing the shoes.

Physical findings
There is prominence of the fifth metatarsal head laterally, usually associated with some medial angulation (varus) of the fifth toe, which sometimes underlaps the fourth toe. Careful palpation can identify tenderness over the prominent fifth metatarsal head; often, there is bursal swelling in this area. The skin shows a tender callus laterally, plantarly, or plantar laterally at the level of the fifth metatarsal head. The deformity is accentuated with weight bearing, and the forefoot is frequently splayed.

Imaging and laboratory studies
A standing anteroposterior radiograph of the forefoot shows prominence of the fifth metatarsal head and perhaps varus angulation of the little toe at the metatarsophalangeal joint. In addition, lateral bowing of the fifth metatarsal may be present, or the fifth metatarsal head may be larger than normal (Fig. 1).

Complications
In diabetic patients or other patients with loss of protective sensation, a blister or pressure sore may develop over the prominent bunionette, resulting in chronic ulceration.

Differential diagnosis
Other causes of metatarsalgia should be considered: Morton's neuroma, arthritis of the fifth metatarsophalangeal joint, and a painful interdigital corn in the fourth web space.

Etiology or pathophysiology
Persistent pain over a prominent bunionette is almost always caused by shoewear that is too tight. The tight shoe compresses the metatarsal heads together, applying direct pressure over the lateral aspect of the fifth metatarsal head. A painful bursa develops to protect the metatarsal head from the shoe pressure, and a tender callus develops to protect the toe from the mechanical irritation of the shoe. The problem is accentuated by lateral bowing of the fifth metatarsal or abnormal widening of the intermetatarsal angle between the fourth and fifth rays.

Epidemiology
This problem is more common in patients who wear high-heeled, pointed-toed shoes and boots and patients whose occupation involves long-term application of pressure to the lateral border of the fifth metatarsal (eg, tailors, who sit on the floor for long hours with their legs crossed at the ankles).

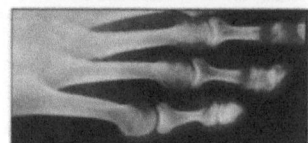

Figure 1. Radiograph of a bunionette.

Treatment

Nonsurgical

The first step in the management of this problem is to have the patient wear shoes with an adequately sized toe box to accommodate the width and depth of the forefoot. Donut-shaped bunion pads can be applied over the bunionette to distribute shoe pressure around the periphery of the metatarsal head and relieve direct pressure. Direct pressure over the metatarsal head should be prevented by avoiding sitting on the floor with legs crossed at the ankles.

Surgical

Surgery should be reserved for the failure of nonsurgical treatment. It is directed at removing the bony prominence of the fifth metatarsal head by 1) removal of the prominence of the plantar and lateral aspects of the fifth metatarsal head or 2) one of several osteotomies of the shaft of the fifth metatarsal designed to shift the fifth metatarsal head medially and dorsally. These operations make the lateral aspect of the fifth metatarsal head less prominent and transfer some of the weight-bearing pressure to the fourth metatarsal head. Recalcitrant pain or recurrent ulcerations can be treated with resection of the entire fifth metatarsal head.

Exercise and activity modification

Shoewear modification is the key to the initial treatment of symptomatic bunionette and usually relieves the symptoms.·

Treatment aims
To relieve the pain and excessive pressure overlying the fifth metatarsal head and transfer weight-bearing pressures to other parts of the forefoot.

Prognosis
Generally the prognosis is good for patients who modify their shoewear. Recalcitrant problems usually respond well to surgical treatment.

Follow-up and management
Shoewear must be carefully selected or the symptomatic bunionette will recur.

Key references
1. Coughlin MJ: Etiology and treatment of the bunionette deformity. In: *Instructional Course Lectures* vol 36. Edited by Greene WB. Rosemont, IL: American Academy of Orthopaedic Surgeons; 1990:37–48.
2. Thompson FM, Coughlin MJ: The high price of high fashion footwear. *J Bone Joint Surg* 1994, 76A:1586–1593.

Diagnosis

Definition
Pseudogout is a form of arthritis caused by deposits of calcium pyrophosphate dihydrate (CPPD) crystals in joints. The term *pseudogout* refers to the gout-like attacks of joint inflammation that occur in many patients with this condition. *Chondrocalcinosis* is the term used to describe the calcium-containing crystal deposits that are found in cartilage and may be visible on joint radiographs.

History
Acute inflammation develops abruptly and lasts for several days or more; it commonly involves the knee. Although the attack may be as severe as a gouty attack, on average it is usually less painful. Five percent of patients demonstrate multiple joint involvement. Pseudogout may be precipitated by surgery or illness. Symptom onset in pseudogout is usually more insidious than in gout and may occur over a period of several days.

Physical findings
Hot swollen joints are noted during an acute attack, often about the knee. Five percent of patients may demonstrate multiple, symmetric joint involvement mimicking rheumatoid arthritis. Weight-bearing joints progressively degenerate.

Imaging and laboratory studies
Radiographs show punctate and linear densities in articular cartilage.

Joint aspirate shows rod-like CPPD crystals positively birefringent when using a polarizing microscope.

Complications
Progressive arthritis.

Flexion contractures.

Charcot arthropathy.

Differential diagnosis
Gout.
Rheumatoid arthritis.
Septic arthritis.

Etiology or pathophysiology
Pseudogout results from the abnormal formation of CPPD crystals in the cartilage. This is followed by the release of crystals into the synovial fluid. When CPPD crystals are released into the joint, they can cause a sudden attack of arthritis similar to gout.
The cause of abnormal deposits of CPP crystals in cartilage is unknown. They may form as a result of abnormal properties of cells in the cartilage, or they may be produced from another disease that damages cartilage. The crystals may be released from cartilage during a sudden illness, joint injury, or previous surgery. The abnormal formation of CPPD crystals may also be a hereditary trait.

Classification
Hereditary.
Idiopathic (increases with age).
Associated with metabolic disease.
Associated with joint trauma.

Epidemiology
Pseudogout is common, especially among older persons. The prevalence is about 3% among people in their 60s and increases with each subsequent decade to as high as 50% in people older than 90 years of age.
Pseudogout affects both men and women. The male-to-female ratio is 1.5:1. Patients with a thyroid condition, kidney failure, or disorders that affect calcium, phosphate, or iron metabolism have an increased risk for pseudogout.
Pseudogout is also common in patients with osteoarthritis, and "attacks" of osteoarthritis associated with pain, swelling, and redness of the joint may in fact be due to pseudogout.
Pseudogout in young patients is unusual. Its occurrence should lead the physician to look for metabolic and hereditary disorders.

Treatment

Nonsurgical
Nonsteroidal anti-inflammatory drugs for the acute attack or colchicine are sometimes given. Intra-articular steroids may be given for acute relief or for those patients unable to tolerate nonsteroidal anti-inflammatory drugs.

Surgical
Arthrocentesis relieves the pressure of accumulated synovial fluid and provides material for diagnosis.

Exercise and activity modification
The affected joint should be splinted for comfort. Crutches may be used as needed.

Treatment aims
To reduce inflammation.

Prognosis
Pseudogout usually is self-limiting and heals well.

Follow-up and management
Follow-up care should be performed as symptoms dictate.

Key references
1. Schumacher HR: *Primer on the Rheumatic Diseases* edn 10. Atlanta: The Arthritis Foundation; 1993.

31

Diagnosis

History
Dropping things.

Chronic repetitive activities (*eg*, computer work, knitting).

Previous wrist fractures.

Physical findings
Numbness in hand in median nerve distribution.

Numbness that awakens patient at night.

Tinel's sign at the wrist (tapping on volar surface of wrist causes paresthesias in median nerve distribution).

Phalen's sign (marked wrist flexion causes median nerve paresthesias).

Decreased sensation to two points in median nerve distribution.

Atrophy of thenar muscles.

Imaging and laboratory studies
Nerve conduction studies reveal slowing of nerve conduction velocity over carpal tunnel.

Electromyography may show denervation in thenar muscles.

Complications
Loss of motor function in thenar muscle group.

Permanent sensory dysfunction in median distribution.

Reflex dystrophy.

Differential diagnosis
Cervical disk disease.

Median nerve entrapment proximally in arm or forearm.

Peripheral neuropathy secondary to diabetes or other endocrinologic cause.

Etiology or pathophysiology
Disorder may affect both hands.

Other nerve entrapment may be associated, eg, cubital tunnel syndrome.

May be associated with trigger finger, de Quervain's syndrome, or rheumatoid arthritis.

Acute carpal tunnel syndrome may be associated with trauma.

Tenosynovitis of flexor tendons at the wrist compromises the cross-sectional area of the carpal tunnel.

Malunion of Colles fracture causes late carpal tunnel syndrome.

Treatment

Nonsurgical
Nonsteroidal anti-inflammatory drugs.
Steroid injection into carpal tunnel.
Night splint with wrist supported in neutral position.

Surgical
Carpal tunnel release at surgery.

Exercise and activity modification
Volar splints, occupational changes, ergonomics, exercise.

Treatment aims
To decrease pain and discomfort.
To preserve muscle function.
To preserve sensation.

Prognosis
40% to 50% of patients improve with nonsurgical treatment.
70% to 80% of patients improve after surgery.
Recurrence after successful surgery is rare.

Follow-up and management
Postsurgical follow-up should include scar massage and exercise for strengthening and to improve motor skills.

Key references
1. Agee JM, McCarroll HR Jr, Tortosa R, et al.
2. Endoscopic release of the carpal tunnel: a randomized prospective multicenter study. J Hand Surg 1992, 17A:987–995.
3. Cobb TK, Amadio PC, et al.: Outcome of reoperation for carpal tunnel syndrome. J Hand Surg 1996, 21A:347–356.
4. Durkan JA: A new diagnostic test for carpal tunnel syndrome. J Bone Joint Surg 1991, 73A:535–538.
5. Grundberg AB: Carpal tunnel decompression in spite of normal electromyography. J Hand Surg 1983, 8:348–349.
6. Levine DW, Simmons BP, Koris MJ, et al.: A self-administered questionnaire for the assessment of severity of symptoms and functional status in carpal tunnel syndrome. J Bone Joint Surg 1993, 75A:1585–1592.

Diagnosis

History

Pain: most patients experience neck, shoulder, and arm pain in varying ratios. Occipital headache is not uncommon. Symptoms often correlate with various head positions, particularly neck hyperextension.

Paresthesias and numbness: sensory abnormalities are highly variable and often do not follow a specific dermatomal pattern. Approximately 50% of patients with nerve root compression have symptoms in a strict radicular pattern. Complete sensory loss in one or more dermatomes is common.

Weakness: shoulder and arm musculature primary involvement is present in 60% to 70% of patients with radiculopathy. Weakness may be found in the lower extremity in cases of spinal cord compression (myelopathy).

Physical Findings

Muscle atrophy: usually found in the shoulder and arm.

Sensory loss: loss of perception in the lateral neck and shoulder (C4 nerve root), lateral arm (C5), lateral forearm, thumb, and index finger (C6), middle finger (C7), ulnar hand (C8) and ulnar forearm (T1).

Motor loss: decreased function in the deltoid muscle (C5 nerve root), biceps, and wrist extensors (C6), triceps and wrist flexors (C7), finger flexors and interosseous muscles (C8), and interossei alone (T1).

Myelopathy: pathologic or functional changes in the spinal cord are indicative of cord compression. Symptoms may include weakness, sensory loss, proprioception loss, and atrophy. Primary signs (upper motor neurologic findings) are clonus, hyperreflexia, Babinski's sign, Hoffman's sign, and inverted radial reflex (ipsilateral finger flexion with brachioradialis reflex).

Imaging and laboratory studies

Plain radiography: the initial diagnostic study should include anteroposterior (AP), lateral, flexion and extension, and oblique views. Degenerative changes on radiographs often do not correlate with symptoms. Radiographs should be examined for facet joint changes, osteophytes, and disk space narrowing. Flexion and extension views can demonstrate cervical instability. Oblique views can show narrowing of the neuroforamina.

Magnetic resonance imaging: T1- and T2-weighted sequences provide evaluation of intraspinal and extraspinal disorders, and of nerve root anatomy. Magnetic resonance imaging (MRI) shows compressive pathology well (Fig. 1). Correlation the patient's history with a physical examination is imperative because of the high number of false positive MRI scans.

Myelography: cervical myelograms outline the spinal cord and exiting nerve roots well. Myelography is a less attractive study because of the delay in visualization, the dilution of dye for cervical imaging, and risk of dye passage into foramen magnum.

Computed tomography myelography: in preoperative planning or in cases of a nonspecific MRI study, Computed tomography myelography is useful; however, it has not been shown to be superior to MRI in evaluating cervical radiculopathy.

Electrodiagnosis: although electrodiagnosis has a high false-negative rate it is useful in differentiating peripheral nerve compression or entrapment from more central compressive process.

Complications

Persistent pain.

Progressive motor sensory deficit.

Myelopathy.

Treatment

Nonsurgical

Most cases of cervical radiculopathy, with the exception of a severe or progressive neurologic deficit, cases of compression secondary to infection, tumor, or cervical spine trauma can initially be managed nonoperatively. The initial treatment regimen depends upon the severity of symptoms and specific pathologic process involved. For acute neck pain and muscle spasm, treatment may include rest, immobilization, local modalities (ice, heat, massage, and electrical stimulation), traction, and anti-inflammatory and antispasmodic agents.

Immobilization: activity modification and temporary use of a soft collar are often used. Immobilization in a position of comfort decreases the acute inflammatory response, muscle spasms, and pain. A short course of bed rest may also be beneficial. An inverted-V pillow may help to relieve radicular symptoms. Home traction devices (8 to 12 lb for 15 to 20 min) provide relief for some patients.

Pharmacologic: narcotic medication may be used initially for acute severe discomfort. Nonsteroidal anti-inflammatory drugs decrease pain caused by the acute inflammatory process. Oral corticosteroids have been shown to reduce nerve root injury if administered in the first 24 to 48 hours but are controversial because of associated side effects. Epidural steroids currently are highly recommended for patients with cervical radiculopathy. Repeat injections may be necessary to continue the anti-inflammatory effects of epidural agents.

Surgical

Indications for surgery include myelopathy with neurologic deficit or a severe or persistent radiculopathy with pain and weakness. Surgery for isolated neck pain secondary to disk disease is less successful. For cases of a single level, posterolateral soft disk herniation, a posterior foraminotomy is useful. More extensive degenerative disease that involves one or more levels may require an anterior diskectomy and block fusion with bone graft, fibular graft, or allograft. Multilevel spondylosis with impingement or myelopathy requires a more aggressive surgical treatment regimen. Anterior vertebrectomies with strut graft placement can be used. Multilevel posterior laminectomy and decompression may fail because of inadequate anterior decompression or progressive kyphosis.

Exercise and activity modification

Patients should avoid aggravating activities. Rest and immobilization are recommended initially. Patients may progress to stretching and strengthening exercises when acute pain and spasms are controlled.

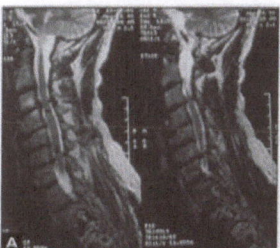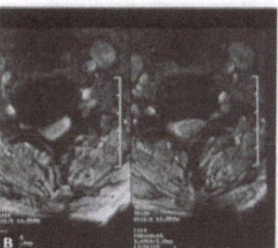

Figure 1. A, Sagittal T1-weighted magnetic resonance imaging (MRI) with herniated nucleus pulposus (HNP) at C3-4 and C6-7. Figure shows levels of compression. B, Axial MRI with HNP at C6-7. Figure shows neural elements compressed by herniation of the nucleus pulposus (HNP).

Treatment aims
To alleviate discomfort and to return patients to an active asymptomatic lifestyle.

Prognosis
Approximately 90% of patients who are treated nonoperatively recover and are asymptomatic.

Key references

1. Bernhardt MH, Hynes RA, Blume HW, et al: Cervical spondylotic myelopathy. *J Bone Joint Surg* 1993, 75A:119–130.

2. Bohlman HH, Emery SE, Goodfellow PB, et al: Robinson anterior cervical discectomy and arthrodesis for cervical radiculopathy. *J Bone Joint Surg* 1993, 75A:1298–1307.

3. Levine MJ, Albert TJ, Smith MD: Cervical radiculopathy: diagnosis and nonoperative management. *J Am Acad Orthop Surg* 1996, 4:305–316.

4. Robinson RA, Smith GW: Anterior lateral cervical disc removal in interbody fusion for cervical disc disease. *Bull Johns Hopkins Hosp* 1955, 96:223–224.

5. Smith GW, Robinson RA: The treatment of certain cervical spine disorders by anterior removal of the intervertebral disk and interbody fusion. *J Bone Joint Surg* 1958, 40:607–623.

A. Agarwal

Diagnosis

History
Most patients with cervical spine fractures have been involved in motor vehicle collisions or falls from significant heights. All trauma patients should be treated as if they have a cervical spine fracture until such a fracture is disproved.

Physical findings
Patients with cervical spine fractures may have neck pain and tenderness to palpation over the spinous process. Neurologic findings may be present depending on the type of injury and its severity. A thorough physical examination that includes a complete neurologic evaluation is indicated. Reflexes to test include the biceps (C5 to C6), triceps (C7), and brachioradialis (C6). Many patients have associated fascial injuries, which should arouse suspicion for a concomitant cervical spine injury.

The neck must be palpated, and step-off or tenderness to palpation should be assessed. Rectal tone must be documented. In cases of suspected spinal shock, bulbocavernosus reflex should be checked and properly documented. The absence of the reflex indicates spinal shock. The return of the reflex signifies the end of spinal shock.

A complete trauma work-up is indicated; the basics must be adhered to. Vital signs indicating neurogenic shock must be addressed. This state of relative hypotension results from a loss of sympathetic tone with unopposed vagal parasympathetic vasodilatation. The hallmark of neurogenic shock is bradycardia despite the hypotension. If tachycardia is present, another source for the hypotension should be sought.

Imaging and laboratory studies
The initial radiographic evaluation of the cervical spine in a trauma patient is usually the lateral; this is the most important imaging study (Fig. 1). Approximately 85% of injuries can be detected with this one view. All cervical levels to the top of T1 should be visualized on the lateral view. If this is not possible, a swimmer's view must be performed (Fig. 2). Once lateral radiography is performed and the patient has undergone the initial survey, an anteroposterior (Fig. 3) and open-mouth (Fig. 4) view should be added for completeness. Oblique views are rarely indicated in the patient suspected of a cervical spine fracture, although isolated fractures of the pedicle, articular mass, or facet joint can be better visualized when other views are negative. Flexion-extension views should be avoided in acute trauma cases but are valuable in the patient who has normal radiographs and continued pain 1 to 2 weeks after the acute trauma. These special views detect ligamentous instability.

Computed tomography remains the best study with which to examine traumatic bony lesions of the cervical spine (Fig. 5). Sagittal and coronal reconstructions are extremely helpful as well (Fig. 6). Magnetic resonance imaging (MRI) is useful in the patient who has normal radiographs but also has pain or a neurologic deficit. Many authors have recommended MRI in cases of facet dislocations for assessment of the status of the intervertebral disk before and after reduction. This is especially true in the case of a bilateral facet dislocation in a neurologically intact patient. Cord injuries without bony injury can also be detected.

Complications
Failure to diagnose a cervical spine injury can be disastrous. It can lead to subsequent neurologic injury, instability, and deformity. The major complication is quadriplegia. Patients with spinal cord injury can also subsequently suffer from other complications.

Differential diagnosis
Primary differential diagnoses are whiplash injury or a ligamentous injury. The radiographs in these cases are usually normal.

Etiology or pathophysiology
Most cervical spine fractures result from high-energy trauma, such as a motor vehicle collision, falls, or diving accidents. The exact mechanical force exerted on the spine can vary. This variation results in several different fracture patterns at all cervical levels.

Neurologic injury can also be classified according to either root or cord involvement. Cord injury is then classified as complete or incomplete. Incomplete cord syndromes are anterior cord syndrome, posterior cord syndrome, central cord syndrome, and Brown-Sequard syndrome.

Epidemiology
Only 20% of fractures have neurologic deficits. Cervical spine fractures are generally divided into injuries of the upper cervical region (C1 or C2) and the sub-axial injuries (C3 and below). Fractures of the atlas (C1) account for 10% of all cervical spine fractures. Moreover, 50% of these patients will also have an associated spine fracture, usually of C2. C1 fractures can involve the anterior or posterior arch or the lateral masses. A fracture of both the anterior and posterior arch, also known as a "burst" fracture, has been called a Jefferson fracture. Fractures of the axis (C2) involve either the dens (odontoid) or the pars interarticularis, resulting in traumatic spondylolisthesis of C2. Of all cervical spine fractures, 15% are odontoid fractures; these are among the most commonly missed spinal injuries. Classification is divided into three types. Type I fracture is a fracture through the tip of the dens and is extremely rare. Type II fracture occurs at the base of the odontoid and is the most common fracture type. Type III fracture extends into the body of C2. A fracture through the pars on both sides results in traumatic spondylolisthesis of the C2 on C3. This has been historically referred to as the "hangman's" fracture. The modern classification, by Levine, has four types. Type I injuries are nondisplaced or have up to 3 mm of displacement but no angulation, and they result from a hyperextension-axial load

(Continued)

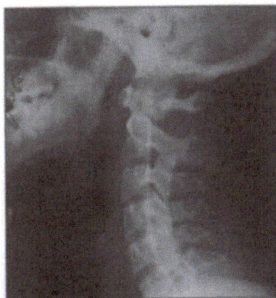

Figure 1. Lateral radiograph of a patient who experienced trauma. Note the inability of the physician to see below C6.

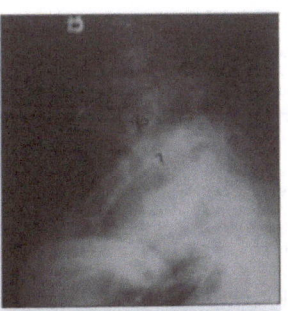

Figure 2. Swimmer's view of the patient shown in Figure 1. The radiograph does show C7, which indicates a fracture of the vertebral body.

Epidemiology

mechanism. The Type II fracture has displacement and angulation resulting from a hyperextension-axial load combined with rebound flexion. The Type IIA fracture has displacement and angulation with varying degrees of severity, but it occurs from a flexion-distraction mechanism. The Type III fracture, which is extremely rare, has an associated unilateral or bilateral facet dislocation in addition to the fracture of the posterior elements. This occurs from a flexion-compression force.

The subaxial cervical spine fractures include the C3-C7 levels. Allen and Ferguson have devised a mechanistic classification for these fractures. This classification is based on the position of the neck at the time of injury and the dominant mode of force application. These are compressive flexion (stages I through V), vertical compression (stages I through III), distractive flexion (stages I through IV), compressive extension (stages I through V), distractive extension (stages I through II), and lateral flexion (stages I through II). The distractive-flexion injury is the most common.

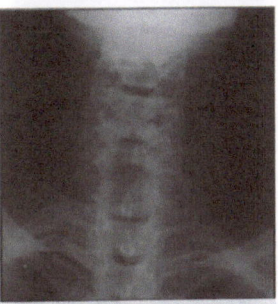

Figure 3. An anteroposterior (AP) radiograph of the patient shown in Figure 1.

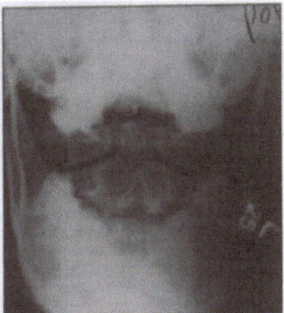

Figure 4. An open-mouth view of the patient shown in Figure 1.

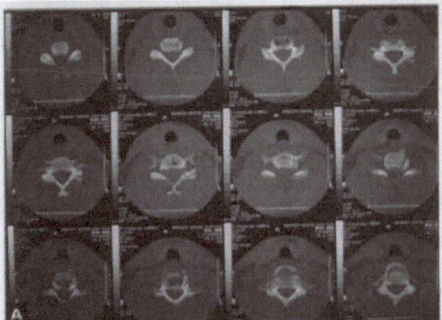

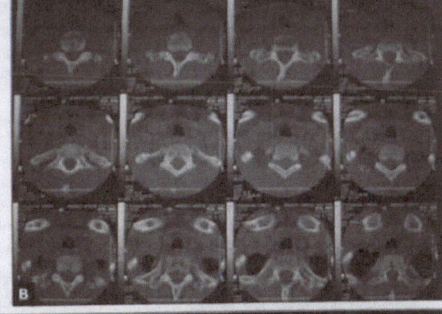

Figure 5. CT scans of the C7 fracture. Axial cuts of C5-T2 are shown. The slices can be followed from A, C5-7 to B, C7-T2. The fracture lines of the body of C7 can be seen easily in the cuts.

Treatment

Nonsurgical

Most C1 fractures can be treated with rigid cervical immobilization for 8 to 12 weeks. The Jefferson fracture is best treated with a halo. The treatment of odontoid fractures varies with the type. Type I fractures can be treated with a Philadelphia collar, and Type III fractures have a high union rate with halo vest immobilization.

Traumatic spondylolisthesis of the axis (Fig. 7) is treated with halo vest immobilization for 8 weeks, followed by 4 weeks of a rigid cervical orthosis. Nonoperative treatment of subaxial injuries usually requires rigid cervical immobilization, generally for about 8 to 12 weeks. A rigid cervical collar is often used, but in some cases a halo is needed. Most types of cervical injuries, all stage I and some stage II, can be treated with a rigid cervical orthosis or halo for 8 to 12 weeks:

Compression flexion injuries, stages I and II.

Vertical compression fractures, stages I and II.

Compression extension fractures, stages I and II.

Distractive extension fractures, stage I.

Lateral flexion fractures, stage I.

Surgical

All patients exhibiting neurologic injury who present within 8 hours of the injury should receive steroids according to the National Acute Spinal Cord Injury Study protocol by Bracken. This entails giving the patient a corticosteroid bolus of 30 mg/kg of body weight, followed by a corticosteroid infusion of 5.4 mg/kg/h for 23 hours. Efficacy has been shown only for blunt cord injuries; this steroid treatment is not indicated for pure root injuries.

The treatment of such injuries is extremely complex and varies with the level and type of injury. In general, unstable injuries require surgical stabilization. Surgical decompression is indicated for all cases of demonstrable neurologic compression, despite realignment of the spine, with a neurologic deficit. The site of neurologic compression directs the surgical approach. Most often, the offending structure is the intervertebral disk; thus, an anterior approach is most often used. Laminectomy is controversial because it tends to predispose the patient to a late kyphotic deformity. A dual approach, anterior and posterior, is sometimes needed for optimum treatment.

Type II odontoid fractures have the highest rate of nonunion with halo immobilization; therefore, many physicians have turned toward anterior screw fixation as an alternative.

The operative treatment of subaxial injuries is usually reserved for the more severe cervical injuries, usually stage II and higher. All distractive flexion injuries require surgical stabilization. The following injuries require surgical intervention:

Compression flexion fractures, stage III: halo vest plus posterior fusion.

Compression flexion fractures, stage IV and V: anterior decompression and strut-graft reconstruction, with or without internal fixation, plus posterior fusion and postoperative halo immobilization.

Vertical compression fractures, stage III: anterior corpectomy and reconstruction, with or without posterior fusion.

Distractive flexion fractures, stages I through IV: closed reduction attempted, followed by open reduction if closed reduction fails, plus primary posterior cervical fusion.

Compression extension fractures, stages III, IV, and V: anterior fusion.

Distractive extension fractures, stage II: anterior fusion with plate fixation.

Lateral flexion fractures, stage II: surgical stabilization and fusion.

(Continued)

Treatment aims

The general goals in the treatment of these injuries are the same for both surgical and nonsurgical management: restoring alignment and stability of the spine while restoring and protecting neurologic function. Internal fixation devices allow reduction, stabilization, early mobilization, decreased hospital stay, and the prevention of pain and deformity.

Prognosis

The prognosis of cervical spine fractures varies according to the type and severity of injury. The main prognostic factor is whether a neurologic deficit is present and whether it is complete or incomplete. Steroid protocol has been shown to improve the neurologic outcome of patients with cord injuries. Approximately 75% of patients with central cord syndromes have functional motor recovery, whereas only 10% with an anterior cord injury have any functional recovery. Brown-Sequard syndrome is associated with the best prognosis; more than 90% of these patients have some functional motor recovery.

Follow-up and management

All patients need long-term follow-up. Management of patients with spinal cord injury should be multidisciplinary, and should include social workers and physical medicine and rehabilitation physicians. Surgical patients still require bracing postoperatively for approximately 8 to 12 weeks. Muscle tone and joint mobility should be maintained as best as possible, especially in paraplegic patients. Self-catheterization should be taught to patients with bladder dysfunction. Once the fracture has healed and the patient no longer needs a brace, physical therapy should initiated in patients who are able.

Key references

1. An HS: Cervical spine trauma. *Spine* 1998, 23:2713–2729.

2. Rizzolo SJ, Cotler JM: Unstable cervical spine injuries: specific treatment approaches. *J Am Acad Orthop Surg* 1993, 1:57–66.

Exercise and activity modification

The patient is restricted from strenuous activity until the fracture has healed; this generally takes 3 months. Time to healing varies, however, according to the injury and the patient. The decision to allow the patient to return to athletic activities is made on a case-by-case basis, with consideration of the patient's injury.

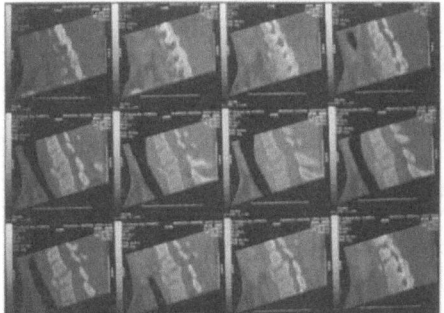

Figure 6. Sagittal reconstructions are important to determine the extent and degree of angular deformity. Note the extent of involvement and the mild kyposis shown in this figure.

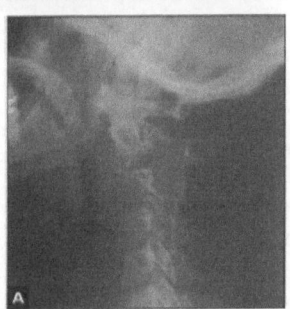

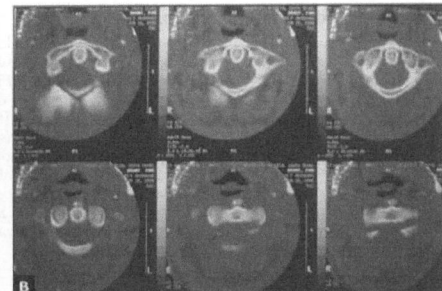

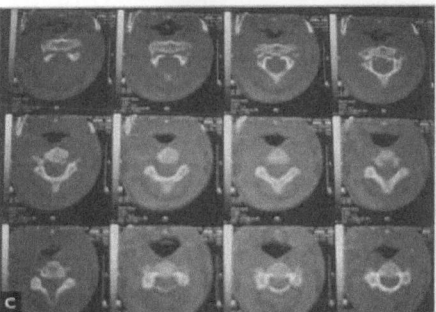

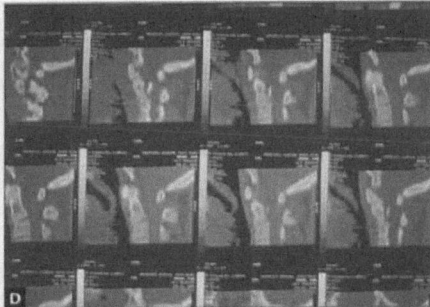

Figure 7. A, Anteroposterior radiograph of a "hangman's" fracture. The fracture of the bilateral pars can be best visualized on the CT scans. B, CT scans of the normal relationship between C1 and C2. C, CT scans of the body of C2 and the fracture lines through the pars. D, CT scans of sagittal reconstruction show the anterior subluxation of C2 on C3.

Diagnosis

History

Patients with cervical spondylosis (degenerative disk disease) usually have a history of insidious onset of neck pain with gradual progression of symptoms. Patients also report associated pain around the shoulders, scapula, and occasionally radicular symptoms of the upper extremities. Pain is also not uncommon in the occipital region. Patients tend to correlate the pain with various head positions, with worse pain in neck hyperextension. If patients have significant radicular symptoms, they may also have motor or sensory abnormalities in the dermatomal distribution of the upper extremities. In severe cases, the patient may complain of upper and lower extremity weakness, sensory changes, and gait abnormalities (myelopathy).

Physical findings

At clinical examination, patients with predominantly cervical spondylosis have pain primarily in the neck, medial scapular region, and shoulder, particularly with hyperextension and rotation of the neck (Spurling's maneuver). If patients have an associated nerve root compression with radiculopathy, clinical examination may reveal upper extremity muscle atrophy, sensory loss, motor weakness, and neck and shoulder pain. Physical examination may reveal a positive clonus, hyperreflexia, and Babinski's sign in patients with cord compression and myelopathy. Mechanical stresses like passive vertebral motion may exacerbate these symptoms.

Imaging and laboratory studies

Initial work-up should consist of plain radiographs in the anteroposterior, lateral, flexion-extension, and oblique views (Fig. 1). Radiographs should be examined for facet joint changes, osteophytes, and disk space narrowing. Flexion-extension views may demonstrate cervical instability. Oblique views may demonstrate narrowing of the neural foramina. Magnetic resonance imaging (MRI) with T1-weighted and T2-weighted sequences permit evaluation of intraspinal, extraspinal disorders, and nerve root anatomy. MRI is highly sensitive for compressive neural pathology. Computed tomography (CT) myelography is useful for preoperative planning of specific neural compressive pathology or in a nonspecific MRI study. However, CT myelography has not been shown to be superior to MRI in evaluating cervical radiculopathy. Electrodiagnosis may also be used for evaluating neural compressive pathology, but it has a high false-negative rate.

Complications

Complications of the anterior approach include neurologic injury, upper airway obstruction, recurrent laryngeal nerve injury, or pseudarthrosis. Complications of laminectomy include subluxation if facet joints are compromised, leading to progressive swan neck deformity and direct spinal cord injury.

Differential diagnosis

Entrapment syndromes of the upper extremity; degenerative joint disease of the shoulder or upper extremity; intraspinal or extraspinal tumor; cervical spine infection; cervical spine fracture; thoracic outlet syndrome; congenital cervical stenosis.

Etiology or pathophysiology

Pathophysiology is the same as degenerative disk disease in other areas of the spine. Chronic disk degeneration and facet arthropathy result in discogenic neck pain and possible neural element compression because the degenerative process involves two facet joints and two uncovertebral joints of Luschka. As a result, progressive canal compromise leads to neural element compression. Progressive stiffening of the cervical spine and loss of motion are an end result of the continued hypertrophic changes.

Epidemiology

Cervical spondylosis typically begins between the ages 40 and 50, with an increased incidence in men by a ratio of 1.4:1. After C5-C6 levels, the C6-C7 levels are most commonly involved. Risk factors are cigarette smoking, heavy lifting on the job, and frequent diving from a board. Patients with cervical disk disease are also more likely to have lumbar disk disease.

Treatment

Nonsurgical

Most cases of discogenic neck pain and radiculopathy can be treated nonsurgically. A combination of nonsteroidal anti-inflammatory drugs (NSAIDs), exercise, immobilization, physical therapy, and, occasionally, cervical traction are beneficial. The initial treatment regimen depends on the severity of symptoms and the specific pathologic process involved. Nonsurgical treatment is less likely to be successful in patients with a severe or progressive neurologic deficit. Narcotic medications may be used initially for acute severe discomfort. NSAIDs can decrease the pain caused by the acute inflammatory process. Oral corticosteroids have been shown to reduce nerve root injury if administered in the first 24 to 48 hours; however, their use is controversial because of the associated side effects. Epidural steroids currently are highly recommended if cervical radiculopathy is present.

Treatment Aim
To alleviate discomfort and to return patients to an active asymptomatic lifestyle

Prognosis
Reported success rates for anterior diskectomy and fusion are greater than 90%.

Surgical

Surgical indications include patients with a severe or progressive cervical radiculopathy or presence of myelopathy. Surgery for isolated neck pain secondary to disk disease is less successful. A posterior foraminotomy may be used for cases of a single-level posterolateral soft disk herniation. More extensive degenerative disease involving one or more levels may require an anterior diskectomy and block fusion with iliac crest bone graft, strut fibular graft, or allograft. Multilevel spondylosis with impingement or myelopathy requires a more extensive surgical treatment regimen. In such a case, multiple anterior vertebrectomies with strut graft placement may be used. Multilevel posterior laminectomy and decompression may fail because of inadequate anterior decompression or progressive kyphosis.

Exercise and activity modification

Patients should avoid aggravating activities. Rest and immobilization are beneficial initially. Therapy with local modalities (eg, ice, heat, and massage) can alleviate pain and muscle spasms. Range-of-motion exercises are encouraged but rapid cervical motion should be avoided.

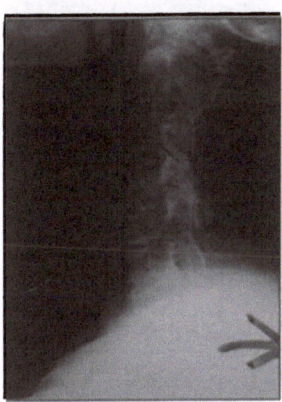

Figure 1. Lateral cervical spine with severe degenerative changes at the C4-5 and C5-6 disk space levels.

Key references
1. Bernhardt M, Hynes RA, Blume HW, et al.: Cervical spondylotic myelopathy. *J Bone Joint Surg* 1993, 75A:119–130.
2. Robinson anterior cervical discectomy and arthrodesis for cervical radiculopathy. *J Bone Joint Surg* 1993, 75A:1298–1307.
3. Cervical radiculopathy: diagnosis and nonoperative management. *J Am Acad Orthop Surg* 1996, 4:305–316.

R.M. Campbell, Jr.

Diagnosis

History

An abused child presents with a fracture or other musculoskeletal injury, and the parents give a false history of injury that is vague, improbable, or nonexistent. As a result, the deliberate nature of the injury is concealed from the physician. Other symptoms of child abuse include delays in seeking medical care for a child's injury, a history of child abuse, and the parents' apparent indifference to the suffering of the child.

Physical findings

Physical signs of swelling and tenderness of a fracture are present, with an explanation that is unreasonable given the severity, location, and type of fracture, eg, a displaced midshaft femur fracture in an infant who "rolled over in bed," an avulsion fracture of the distal humerus from a "touch on the shoulder," and a spiral fracture of a long bone from a direct blow.

Soft tissue injury, such as bruises, welts, scars, and burns, are seen in 80% of abused children. Even in infants, signs of sexual abuse, such as genital or anal bruising or tears, may be present. A tense, tender abdomen suggests blunt abdominal trauma. Infants with altered mental status (shaken baby syndrome) may have occult subdural hematomas with associated retinal bleeding.

Imaging and laboratory studies

Radiographs: anteroposterior and lateral radiographs of the entire long bone are taken to determine location, type, and severity of fracture. No fracture pattern (spiral, transverse, oblique) or location (diaphyseal, metaphyseal, epiphyseal) predominates in child abuse, but the "chip/corner/bucket handle" fracture with a small fragment of metaphysis adjacent to the epiphysis is almost pathognomonic of child abuse (Fig. 1). It is important to objectively estimate the age of fracture: no healing, less than 4 to 10 days; soft callus, 14 to 21 days; hard callus, 21 to 42 days; remodeling present, as early as 3 months. Skeletal survey should always be done and should include anteroposterior and lateral radiographs of the humerus, forearms, femurs, tibias, chest, spine, skull, spine, and anteroposterior of the hands and feet. A "babygram" in lieu of a skeletal survey is not recommended. Oblique chest radiographs can help diagnose subtle rib fractures. Multiple unexplained fractures in different stages of healing are a sign of child abuse.

Other studies: bone scans can visualize occult rib fractures and long bone fractures (Figs. 2 and 3). Computed tomography scans are used to image the acute abdomen and to aid in the diagnosis of subdural hematomas. Clinical photographs are important for documenting soft tissue trauma.

Laboratory studies: complete blood count with erythrocyte sedimentation rate, prothrombin time and partial thromboplastin time, especially with clinical bruising; measurement of amylase levels to rule out pancreatitis; liver function tests (alanine aminotransferase, aspartate aminotransferase, lactate dehydrogenase) to rule out hepatic injury; and drug toxicology when indicated.

Consultations: neurosurgery for altered mental status and ophthalmology to rule out retinal bleeding. Social service consultation can research family situations for economic stress and drug abuse and can determine who has access to the abused child.

Complications

If the child is returned to the abusive environment without intervention, the risk for recurrent serious injury is 25% and the risk for death is 5%.

Differential diagnosis

Osteogenesis imperfecta.
Osteomyelitis.
Copper deficiency syndrome.
Rickets.
Scurvy.
Syphilis.
Septic arthritis.
Leukemia.
Hypophosphatasia.

It is important to carefully document all history and physical findings; incomplete documentation may later be challenged in court. Always ask for family history of metabolic bone disease. Rule out osteogenesis imperfecta by noting bone density on radiography and examining for blue sclera. Equivocal cases of osteogenesis imperfecta may require skin biopsy for fibroblast enzyme assay. Be aware of Münchausen's syndrome by proxy, in which caregivers induce injury or illness in children to provoke unnecessary medical care. Suspicion of child abuse must always be reported to child protective services; failure to do so exposes the physician to misdemeanor penalties and malpractice charges. However, if the evidence does not clearly support a diagnosis of nonaccidental trauma, do not stigmatize the family with the charge of child abuse.

Etiology

Child abuse is more common in single-parent homes; substance abuse situations; and homes threatened by divorce, separation, or loss of job.

Epidemiology

An estimated 1% to 1.5% of all children are abused each year. One child a day dies of child abuse. Orthopedists see 30% to 50% of physical abuse cases.

Treatment

After evaluation, the child is treated for his or her injury and admitted for observation. This places them in a safe environment while the circumstances of injury are investigated and consultations are obtained. If the findings support a diagnosis of child abuse, a notarized affidavit is placed on the chart; this affidavit notes findings, diagnosis of injuries, and the likelihood that they are due to abuse. The child is discharged once child protective services has made a decision about placement.

Treatment aims
To establish a healing environment for both the child and the family, to address the child's injuries with medical care, and to provide a safe place for convalescence with the supervision of child protective services.

Prognosis
With aggressive intervention, the likelihood of repeat child abuse in a family is low.

Follow-up and management
Routine follow-up for injury is coordinated through protective services and may involve supervised visits of the child with parents, family member, or foster parent. The family should be enrolled in any available abuse prevention program.

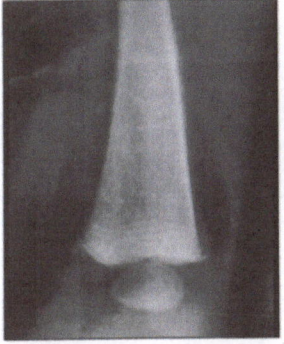

Figure 1. A subtle metaphyseal chip fracture on the distal femur. The fracture is a complete avulsion of the epiphysis, is unique to child abuse, and results from violent shaking of the extremity or from a traction injury. The fracture extends through the radiolucent growth plate exiting from the corner of metaphysis to produce the characteristic chip fracture sign.

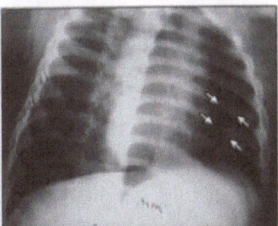

Figure 2. The set of rib fractures associated with acute fracture of the long bone are strongly suggestive of child abuse. Oblique radiographs are helpful in seeing subtle healed rib fractures that appear as fusiform swelling of the ribs (*arrows*).

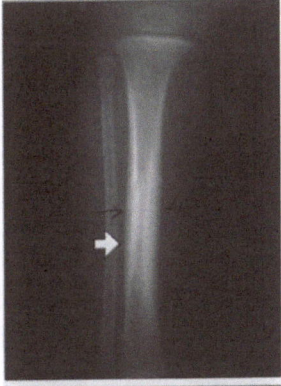

Figure 3. Healed fractures of the long bones in children appear as sclerotic, fusiform thickening of the cortex (*arrow*). Comparison radiographs of the opposite side may be necessary for subtle findings.

Key references
1. Akbarnia BA, Akbarnia NO: The role of the orthopaedist in child abuse and neglect. *Orthop Clin North Am* 1976, 7:773.
2. Campbell RM Jr: *Child Abuse in Special Injuries: Fractures of Children.* Edited by Rockwood CA, Wilkins KE, Beatty J. Philadelphia: JB Lippincott; 1996.

Diagnosis

History

The clavicle is a subcutaneous structure, and displaced fractures of this bone present little difficulty in diagnosis. The history is generally straightforward and reveals some form of indirect or direct injury to the shoulder or chest. Most commonly, the patient reports a fall or blow on the point of the shoulder.

Physical findings

Deformity is usually obvious on visual inspection and may be associated with soft tissue swelling and ecchymosis. In displaced fractures, the proximal fragment is displaced posterosuperiorly, and the skin may be tented. The patient splints the involved extremity at the side to minimize pain associated with movement. Point tenderness is elicited at the fracture site, and the patient tilts his or her head toward the injured side to relax the trapezius muscle.

Imaging and laboratory studies

An anteroposterior view and a 40° to 50° cephalic tilt view are usually obtained for evaluation of clavicle fractures.

Complications

Nonunion and neurovascular sequelae are the most common complications of clavicle fractures. The incidence of nonunion of unoperated shaft fractures is 1% to 4%, and this condition is related to the severity of trauma, the location of the fracture, and the degree of initial displacement. Neurovascular injuries are rare, but brachial plexus neuropraxia, aneurysm, thrombosis, and arterial lacerations have been reported.

Differential diagnosis

Acromioclavicular sprain or dislocation.
Sternoclavicular sprain or dislocation.
Coracoid fracture.
Upper anterior rib fracture.

Etiology or pathophysiology

Clavicle fractures occur by a direct blow to the clavicle or by indirect means, such as a fall on the outstretched hand.

Epidemiology

Clavicle fractures are common in childhood; approximately half of these fractures occur in children 7 years of age or younger. The incidence of clavicle fractures in adults appears to be increasing and has been attributed to an increase in high-velocity motor vehicle injuries and a rising interest in recreational sports. One in 20 fractures occurs in the clavicle.

Treatment

Nonsurgical

In most clavicle fractures, excellent results are obtained with nonsurgical treatment. The goal of nonsurgical treatment is to provide comfortable support of the involved extremity during anticipated healing of the fractured clavicle. Although deformity and shortening usually occur, dysfunction and weakness are rare. Commonly accepted methods of nonsurgical treatment include a simple sling, sling and swathe, a Velpeau dressing, or a commercial figure eight splint.

Surgical

The indications for surgical management of clavicle shaft fractures include open fractures of the clavicle, associated neurovascular injury with ongoing compromise, associated fractures of the scapula that result in an unstable shoulder girdle, and symptomatic nonunions of the clavicle. Effective means of surgical treatment include open reduction and internal fixation with the use of plates, as described by the AO/ASIF group, or intramedullary pin fixation, as described by Boehme.

Treatment aims
To support the upper extremity, allow function of the ipsilateral elbow, wrist, and hand, and achieve fracture healing.

Prognosis
Motion returns by 6 to 8 weeks. Strength and function are usually normal by 3 months.

Follow-up and management (or rehabilitation)
Patients are started on active and passive range-of-motion exercises the day after surgery. Strengthening exercises begin at 6 weeks, with patients returning to most of their activities in 3 months.

Key references

1. Boehme D, Curtis RJ, DeHaan JT, et al.: Non-union of fractures of the midshaft of the clavicle: treatment with a modified Hagie intramedullary and autogenous bone grafting. *J Bone Joint Surg* 1991, 73A:1219–1226.

2. Neer CS II: Fractures of the clavicle. In *Fractures in Adults*. Edited by Rockwood CA Jr, Green DP. Philadelphia: JB Lippincott; 1984:707–713.

3. Rowe CR: An atlas of anatomy and treatment of midclavicular fractures. *Clin Orthop* 1968, 58:29–42.

4. Rüedi T, Schweiberer L: Clavicular fractures (including luxation of adjacent joints). In *Manual of Internal Fixation: Techniques Recommended by the AO-ASIF Group* edn 3. Edited by Müller ME, Allgöwer M, Schneider R, et al. Berlin: Springer-Verlag; 1991:434–435.

Diagnosis

History

Cubital tunnel syndrome is a compressive syndrome of the ulnar nerve at the elbow. Ulnar neuropathy presents with intermittent paresthesias or dysesthesias in the ulnar aspect of the hand and in the small and ring fingers. In the long-standing or chronic state, patients often report constant pain, numbness in the small and ring fingers, clumsiness, and severe weakness. Occupational history frequently reveals that the patient performs duties with the elbow in a hyperflexed position (eg, working at a computer keyboard that is positioned too high).

Physical findings

Discomfort is elicited by palpation of the cubital tunnel (the area between the medial epicondyle and the olecranon). Tenderness may also be noted in the region of the flexor/pronator origin or along the medial intermuscular septum. A positive Tinel's sign is present with percussion of the cubital tunnel. Chronic cases may reveal atrophy of the hypothenar muscle, clawing of the ulnar two digits, and abduction of the small finger (Wartenberg's sign). A useful provocative test involves hyperflexion of the elbow with reproduction or exacerbation of symptoms within 1 to 2 minutes.

Imaging and laboratory studies

Radiographic studies should include anteroposterior, lateral, and cubital tunnel views (ossification of the medial collateral ligament or ossification in the cubital tunnel may be noted).

Sensory evaluation with Semmes Weinstein monofilaments is a reproducible method of determining sensory function.

Findings on electromyography and nerve conduction velocity testing will be positive in moderate and severe cases (a nerve conduction delay of 10 ms or greater across the elbow confirms the diagnosis).

Complications

Persistent, severe dysesthesias are the most common complication and are associated with significant morbidity.

Reflex sympathetic dystrophy.

Persistent sensory deficit.

Persistent weakness.

Differential diagnosis

C8 radiculopathy.

Thoracic outlet syndrome.

Compression of the ulnar nerve in Guyon's canal at the wrist.

Etiology or pathophysiology

Compression is the primary contributor to chronic compressive neuropathy at the elbow.

The compression effect may be the result of elbow flexion and extension, which requires excursion of the nerve to accommodate full motion of the joint. Traction, friction, and direct trauma are additional mechanisms of injury.

Endocrine abnormalities, such as diabetes mellitus, predispose patients to ulnar neuropathy, because these patients are more susceptible to nerve injury in general.

Epidemiology

Approximately half of patients with cubital tunnel syndrome will improve spontaneously. The syndrome is more common in patients with comorbid conditions, such as diabetes mellitus.

Treatment

Nonsurgical
Conservative treatment consists of activity modification (avoidance of prolonged elbow flexion), nonsteroidal anti-inflammatory drugs, extension splinting at night, and the use of elbow pads for patients who work with the elbow flexed on a hard surface.

Surgical
Surgical treatment consists of five main procedures:

Simple ulnar nerve decompression.

Subcutaneous transposition.

Intramuscular transposition.

Submuscular transposition.

Medial epicondylectomy.

The literature reveals 80% to 90% good results with surgical treatment.

Exercise and activity modification
See Nonsurgical Treatment section.

Treatment aims
Improve function.
Decrease or eliminate symptoms.
Avoid intrinsic muscle atrophy and clawing of ulnar digits.

Prognosis
Nonsurgical treatment of mild intermittent cubital tunnel syndrome produces good results in up to 80% of patients.

Follow-up and management (or rehabilitation)
A supportive, well-padded dressing is used after surgery. Range-of-motion exercises are usually instituted immediately, but these exercises may be delayed 1 to 2 weeks when a transposition or epicondylectomy is performed. Function generally returns within 6 months.

Key references
1. Craven PR, Green DP: Cubital tunnel syndrome: treatment by medial epicondylectomy. J Bone Joint Surg 1980, 62A:986–989.
2. James GGH: Nerve lesions about the elbow. J Bone Joint Surg 1956, 38B:589.

Diagnosis

History

Patients with degenerative lumbar disk disease generally will have a history of insidious onset of low back pain with activity. Patients may have experienced acute severe exacerbation of pain that radiates to the buttocks and lower extremities. For isolated degenerative lumbar disk disease without herniated disk, patients will generally have isolated low back pain. In cases of herniated disk, patients may experience back pain, bilateral buttock and lower extremity pain, saddle anesthesia, and possible bowel or bladder dysfunction (urinary retention). Loss of lower extremity motor and sensory function can be variable, depending on the level of the herniated disk. Pain may worsen with standing and sitting, and may be relieved when lying supine or flexing forward.

Physical Findings

At the physical examination, patients should be evaluated for an acute precipitating event. A detailed history should be sought to define the quality and duration of pain. The location of symptoms (especially pain in the lower extremities), nature of the pain, changes with activity, and a thorough review of systems and psychiatric history are useful. Occupational risks should be evaluated for exposure to prolonged walking, sitting, or repetitive lifting activities. Patients should be questioned about constitutional symptoms, any history of night pain, or history of a cancer, which would be suggestive of tumor. At the physical examination, patients should be observed for gait and posture. The examination should include palpation of the spine for tenderness and muscle spasm, assessment of range of motion, rectal examination, vascular evaluation, and neurologic evaluation. Tension signs (straight leg raising, bow string sign, femoral nerve stretch test) are important. These would be indicative of a possible herniated nucleus pulposus (HNP). A positive contralateral straight-leg raise is more specific for an HNP. Inappropriate physical signs and symptoms are important to document. These would include nonorganic physical signs such as tenderness to light touch, pain with light axial loading of the spine, pain with pelvic rotation, negative straight-leg raise while sitting but positive while supine, and nonanatomic dermatomal distribution of symptoms.

Imaging and laboratory investigations

The initial studies should include radiographs in the anterioposterior and lateral planes. Oblique radiographs may be beneficial in cases of a pars defect (spondylolysis) or for evaluation of neuroforamina. Radiographs should be examined for degenerative disk disease, which would include loss of disk space height, sclerosis, osteophytes, and subluxation or spondylolisthesis of the spine (Fig. 1A). Magnetic resonance imaging (MRI) is highly specific and useful for evaluating for a degenerative disk with desiccation (Fig. 1B). Also, MRI is useful for evaluating herniated disk with encroachment on the neural elements and for possible spinal stenosis. Computed tomography (CT) is noninvasive and useful for detecting bony stenosis. When stenosis or compression of the neural foramina is suspected, a myelogram or a postmyelography CT is useful for identifying the areas of encroachment. It should be noted that false-positive MRI scans are common, with a reported 35% false-positive rate in patients less than 40 years of age, and 93% rate in patients more than 60 years of age. Electromyelogphic studies are rarely more beneficial for providing information on neurologic function of the extremities, other than what can be ascertained from a good physical examination.

Complications

Patients with isolated degenerative disk disease without herniated disk may have multilevel involvement with spinal stenosis. Failure to diagnosis stenosis could lead to progressive pain, disability, and neurologic dysfunction. Patients with spondylolisthesis (anterior slip of one vertebra on another) may also have progressive loss of neurologic function in advanced cases. Patients with HNP rarely get chronic pain with permanent loss of neurologic function in the nerve roots affected.

Etiology or pathophysiology

Degenerative disk disease occurs as a normal consequence of aging. Intervertebral disks undergo degenerative changes marked by dehydration of the nucleus pulposus with depletion of proteoglycan content with time. Progressive tearing of annular fibers due to prolonged axial and shear stresses may result in complete tear of the annular ligament. With progressive desiccation of the disk and loss of height, structural integrity of the annular ligament can be compromised with displacement of the nuclear material. Lumbar disk disease often involves the L4-5 disk, followed closely by the L5-S1 level. Most disk herniations occur posterolateral, where the posterior longitudinal ligament is the weakest. Subsequent impingement on the nerve roots thus produces nerve root pain and sciatica. Central prolapse of a disk is usually associated with isolated back pain; however, severe acute central prolapse may result in cauda equina syndrome. Most lumbar disk herniations occur in patients between 30 and 50 years of age. Pathophysiology of sciatic pain involves both mechanical and biochemical factors. It is suspected that inflammatory mediators play a large role in pain syndromes. These include interleukin-1, interleukin-6, nitric oxide, and prostaglandins. The natural history of lumbar disk disease with herniation reveals a more favorable response to conservative treatment, even in the presence of neurologic deficits. Thus, an isolated neurologic deficit does not warrant immediate surgical intervention. Several studies have revealed that a herniated disk, particularly a large extruded herniated disk, will resorb over time.

Epidemiology

The prevalence of disk herniation is complicated by the finding that approximately 35% of patients under the age of 40 who are asymptomatic have herniated disks on MRI. Patients who are more than 60 years of age have approximately 93% prevalence of herniated disk. Estimated lifetime prevalence of symptomatic HNP is approximately 2%. In the United States, surgical intervention is estimated at approximately 160 in 100,000 patients. Given the excellent prognosis in patients with nonsurgical management, many of these operations may be inappropriate.

Treatment

Nonsurgical

The mainstay of treatment for degenerative disk disease with or without herniated disk includes a few days of rest, nonsteroidal anti-inflammatory medications (NSAIDs), physical therapy, and rapid restoration of the patient's ambulating activities. It is estimated that more than 50% of patients with acute low back pain recover in approximately 1 week, and more than 90% recover within 1 to 3 months. More than 50% of patients with sciatica recover within a month. It is important for patients to be sent for physical therapy for back strengthening exercises and for overall aerobic conditioning. Patient education for exacerbating and relieving factors is important as are continuing home exercises. If patients fail to improve within 6 weeks of conservative treatment, then further evaluation is warranted. Patients with a predominance of low back pain should be screened to rule out spinal tumors or infection (bone scan is useful). In patients with HNP, excellent results have been obtained with injection of epidural steroids to decrease inflammation around the nerve roots. This may have to be repeated up to two or three times.

Surgical

Surgical treatment is reserved for patients who have failed conservative treatment or for patients in whom acute cauda equina syndrome develops. The best candidates for surgical diskectomy include patients with a positive physical examination, neurologic findings, positive tension signs with predominantly sciatic symptoms, without any other psychosocial problems. With the proper indications, more than 95% of patients undergoing surgical diskectomy are reported to have initially good or excellent results. It has been reported, however, that as many as 30% of patients may continue to have long-term back pain, even in the presence of complete resolution of lower extremity pain. Complications of surgical intervention for herniated disk include vascular injury, nerve root injury, repeat disk herniation (inadequate decompression), dural tear, infection, and postoperative hematoma. Degenerative lumbar disk disease may also be associated with lumbar segmental instability. A combination of damage to the annulus fibrosus and disk space narrowing may reduce the disk's ability to resist rotation. A continuing degenerative process results in facet subluxation and instability. On dynamic views, angular changes greater than 10° on flexion films and translation of greater than 3–4 mm are characteristic of instability. Surgical treatment options for instability include posterolateral fusion, posterior lumbar interbody fusion, and anterior interbody fusion. Patients may also require internal fixation using pedicle screws and a plate or rod construct. Degenerative disk disease may also be associated with spinal stenosis and spondylolisthesis, which may require surgical intervention (*see* Spinal Stenosis and Spondylolisthesis).

Treatment aims
To achieve reduction in the patient's discomfort and to return the patient to a normal, active lifestyle. The goal of treatment in patients with neurologic deficit is to reduce further neurologic sequelae.

Prognosis
Approximately 90% of properly selected patients undergoing open diskectomy through a limited laminotomy experience successful short-term relief of symptoms. Long-term studies in these patients, however, reveal a progressive decline in the success, resulting from subsequent degenerative changes. Risk of recurrent disk herniation is reported between 5% and 10%. Long-term prognosis for patients with degenerative disk disease and instability who undergo internal fixation are less satisfactory than simple diskectomy.

Follow-up and management
All patients with degenerative lumbar disk disease and sciatica should be followed for progressive symptoms and neurologic deficit. Patients should be on a continuous regimen of NSAIDs and physical therapy for overall aerobic conditioning and back strengthening exercises.

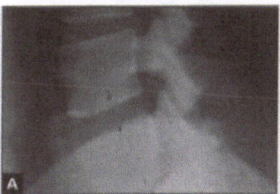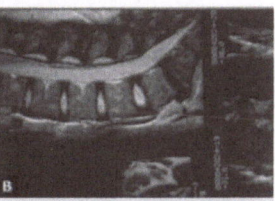

Figure 1. A, Lateral radiograph of a patient with degenerative disk disease at L5-S1. The radiograph shows significant loss of disk height compared with other levels with degenerative changes. B, Magnetic resonance imaging in the same patient with evidence of decreased disk height and desiccation of the disk (*black disk*).

Key references
1. Bell GR, Rothman RH: The conservative treatment of sciatica. Spine 1984, 9:54–56.
2. Kostuik JP, Harrington I, Alexander D, et al: Cauda equina syndrome and lumbar disc herniation. J Bone Joint Surg [Am] 1986, 68:386–391.
3. Waddell G, McCulloch JA, Kummel ED, et al: Failed lumbar disc surgery and repeat surgery following industrial injuries. J Bone Joint Surg 1979, 61A:201–207.
4. Weber H: Lumbar disc herniation: a controlled prospective study with 10 years of observation. Spine 1983, 8:131–140.
5. Lumbar degenerative disc disorders. In Orthopaedic Knowledge Update 6. Edited by Arendt EA. Rosemont, IL: American Orthopaedic Society for Sports Medicine; 1999:685–690.

F.G. Corley

Diagnosis

History
Dorsoradial wrist pain may occur after a fall or trauma. It is often associated with chronic repetitive activities, such as typing.

Physical findings
Swelling over first dorsal compartment.
"Popping" over wrist.
Swelling over wrist.
Tenderness over first dorsal compartment.
Pain on ulnar deviation of the wrist (Finkelstein's test).
Small cyst over first dorsal compartment.
Pain on extension of thumb.

Imaging and laboratory studies
Radiography may reveal swelling over the radial side of the wrist or an exostosis.
Bone scan shows increased uptake over radial wrist.

Complications
Rupture of extensor pollicis brevis.
Rupture of abductor pollicis longus.

Differential diagnosis
Fracture of the scaphoid.
Fracture of the distal radius.
Giant-cell tumor of the distal radius.
Arthritis at the base of the thumb.
Neuroma of superficial branch of the radial nerve.
Aneurysm of radial artery.

Etiology or pathophysiology
Trauma.
Chronic repetitive activity.
Associated with diabetes,
rheumatoid arthritis.
May be associated with carpal tunnel or trigger finger.
Stenosing tenosynovitis of the first dorsal extensor compartment (Fig. 1).

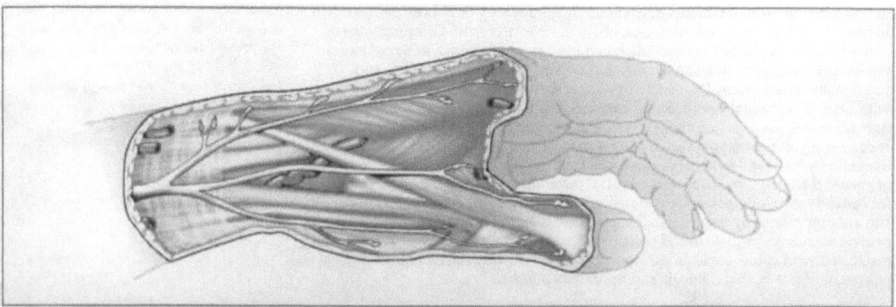

Figure 1. de Quervain's syndrome is a stenosing tenosynovitis of the first dorsal compartment. The first dorsal compartment involves the tendons of the abductor pollicis longus and the extensor pollicis brevis. Other causes of pain in this area are illustrated, including traumatic neuroma of the superficial branches of the radial nerve and possibly arthritis of the base of the thumb (the carpometacarpal joint).

Treatment

Nonsurgical
Nonsteroidal anti-inflammatory drugs given with moist heat and splinting can relieve symptoms acutely.

Steroid injection into the first dorsal compartment can relieve and sometimes cure the syndrome; injections may be given 3 to 4 times a year.

Surgical
Surgical release of the first dorsal compartment under local anesthesia is successful for recalcitrant cases. Complications include painful scar, neuroma, and failure to release all of the compartment.

Exercise and activity modification
No special precautions necessary.

Treatment aims
To lessen inflammation in the compartment and the stenotic component.

Prognosis
With surgery, excellent.

Follow-up and management
At 2 weeks after surgery, suture removal; then massage of scar. Without surgery, steroid injections can be given every 3 to 4 months (Fig. 2).

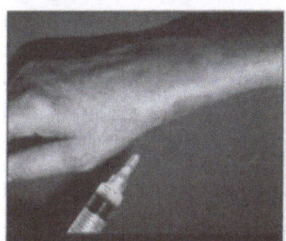

Figure 2. Office treatment of de Quervain's syndrome includes injection of the first dorsal compartment with a steroid local anesthetic solution. A tuberculin hypodermic can be used, and 0.5 mL of Celestone (Schering, Kenilworth, NJ) and 0.5 mL of Xylocaine can easily be introduced into the area of maximal tenderness over the first dorsal compartment. This brings relief in 60% to 80% of these problems.

Key references

1. Chicarilli ZN, Watson HK, Linberg R, Sasaki, G: Saddle deformity. Posttraumatic interosseous-lumbrical adhesions: review of eighty-seven cases. J Hand Surg 1986, 11A:210–218.

2. Grundberg AB, Reagan DS: Pathologic anatomy of the forearm: intersection syndrome. J Hand Surg 1985, 10A:299–302.

3. Lombardi RM, Wood MB, Linscheid RL: Symptomatic restrictive thumb-index flexor tenosynovitis: incidence of musculotendinous anomalies and results of treatment. J Hand Surg 1988, 13A:325–328.

4. Palmieri TJ: Pisiform area pain treatment by pisiform excision. J Hand Surg 1982, 7:477–480.

5. Trumble TE, Watson HK: Posttraumatic sesamoid arthritis of the metacarpophalangeal joint of the thumb. J Hand Surg 1985, 10A:94–100.

Diagnosis

History
Nonambulatory infants have no symptoms of developmental dysplasia. Once they begin walking, children with developmental dislocated hip (DDH) limp without pain. With bilateral disease, children waddle while walking and have excessive lumbar lordosis.

Physical findings
At birth, the affected lower extremity is slightly shortened and sometimes has more skin folds than the other side. With the thighs aligned together and the hips and knees flexed 90°, the involved knee is shorter than the other side; this is a positive result on the Galeazzi test. In frank hip dislocation, the result of the Ortolani test may be positive: the hips are held in 90° of flexion and are gently abducted from neutral, and a "clunk" is felt as the hip reduces at wide abduction. In 15% of infants, a "click" is felt with this maneuver, but this is usually just soft tissue impingement; 5% of "click-positive" infants develop serious hip instability. In a hip that is reduced but is potentially unstable because of acetabular dysplasia, the result of a Barlow test may be positive: the flexed hip is gently pushed posteriorly; subluxation or dislocation of the hip is felt in abnormal hips. Findings on both of these tests may become negative in children with DDH who are older than 2 months; the dislocated hip may become irreducible and an adduction hip contracture may be the only finding at that point.

Imaging and laboratory studies
The standard anteroposterior pelvis-with-hips radiograph is difficult to interpret in the neonatal period because most of the hip is not ossified; however, some radiographic signs are helpful (Figs. 1 and 2). Shenton's line is drawn along the inferior margin of proximal femur and should line up with the inferior margin of the superior pubic ramus of the pelvis in the normal hip. Superior migration of the hip in DDH will disrupt this relationship, causing a "break" in Shenton's line, but subtle instability is hard to see on radiographs. The acetabular index is the angle between a line along the osseous roof of the acetabulum and another line passing through the centers of both acetabulum. It is approximately 30° at birth and reduces to 22° by 2 years of age. Marked differences of the index between hips suggests acetabular dysplasia on the side with an increased index. The appearance of the ossific nucleus of the femoral head is delayed when the hip is unstable. Any hip at risk because of clinical history or suspicious physical findings should undergo assessment by real-time ultrasonography. The infantile cartilaginous hip is easily visualized and shows dislocation and subluxation; in the reduced but unstable hip, ultrasonography also shows acetabular dysplasia. Ultrasonography of the hip is not possible once the ossific nucleus of the hip exceeds 1 cm. Hip arthrography is usually reserved for evaluation of the hips of older children.

Complications
Untreated DDH results in a dislocated, hypoplastic femoral head that rides above a flattened, shallow, true acetabulum to rest against the iliac crest into a false acetabulum. As a result, the lower extremity is shortened, and the altered hip biomechanics leads to a pronounced Trendelenberg limp. Running is difficult, and the hip may become painful later in life. Conversion to a total hip arthroplasty later in adulthood is difficult because of the altered anatomy.

Differential diagnosis
Septic hip.
Fracture of the hip.
Osteomyelitis of femur.
Proximal femoral focal deficiency.

Etiology
The cause is probably a combination of primary acetabular dysplasia, joint laxity, and adverse intrauterine factors (eg, the breech position).

Epidemiology
The incidence of DDH is 1 to 1.5 per 1000 live births. The female-to-male ratio is 4:1. Groups at risk include females with history of breech presentation (1 in 35), firstborn children, infants with a history of oligohydramnios, and family history of DDH. The risk is 6% if a sibling has DDH, 12% if the mother had DDH, and 36% if both the mother and sibling had DDH.

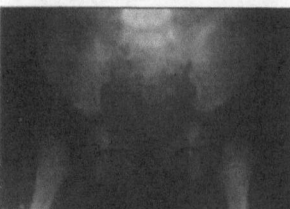

Figure 1. A neonate with bilateral developmental dysplasia of the hip. Shenton's line is broken on the anteroposterior (AP) pelvic radiograph. Note that neither the acetabulum nor the femoral head can be seen on the radiograph at this stage of life.

Treatment

Nonsurgical

From birth to age 6 months, a Pavlik harness brace is applied to the infant to reduce the dislocated hip; it is worn for approximately 6 weeks and successfully stabilizes the hip in 95% of cases. A delay in diagnosis up to 4 weeks of age does not seem to affect the success of brace treatment. Hip ultrasonography is helpful in determining whether the harness has reduced the hip early in treatment and in assessing whether the acetabular dysplasia has resolved adequately to permit brace weaning (Fig. 3).

Surgical

In patients with DDH diagnosed later in life (from older than 6 months through 5 years of age), closed reduction of the hip dislocation with hip adductor myotomy under general anesthesia may be necessary with prolonged casting. Older patients and younger ones not responding to closed treatment may require open operative reduction of the hip. Proximal femoral shortening may be necessary to obtain reduction without excessive femoral head pressure. In an older child, if the acetabulum is dysplastic or the hip is in valgus, an innominate osteotomy of the acetabulum may be needed to augment containment and a varus derotational osteotomy of the hip may be done to center the hip into the depths of the acetabulum.

Prognosis

Early diagnosis and brace treatment will most likely result in a normal hip for the infant with a DDH. Later treatment with casting or operative reduction has a more uncertain prognosis, with the possibility of avascular necrosis of the hip, hip stiffness, postoperative infection, and residual joint instability.

Follow-up and management

Until skeletal maturity, the DDH patient should be followed with physical examination and pelvic radiography.

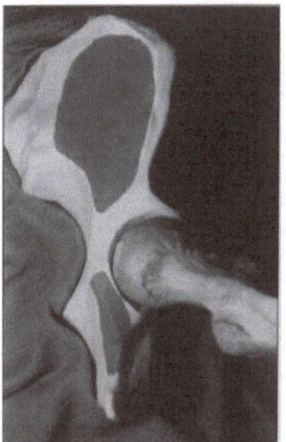

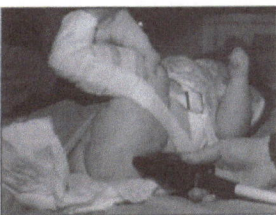

Figure 3. An infant with developmental dysplasia of the hip is being treated with a Pavlik harness. An ultrasound examination determines whether the infant can be weaned from using the harness.

Figure 2. The portion of the neonatal pelvis (grey) that is visible on a radiograph. The acetabulum is primarily cartilage (white). Radiographs, therefore, do not show acetabular dysplasia in this age group.

Key references

1. Barlow TG: Early diagnosis and treatment of congenital dislocation of the hip. J Bone Joint Surg [Br] 1962, 44:292.

2. DeRosa GP, Feller N: Treatment of congenital dislocation of the hip: management before walking age. Clin Orthop 1987, 225:77.

3. Heinrich SD, Missinne LH, MacEwen GD: The conservative management of congenital dislocation of the hip after walking age. Clin Orthop 1992, 281:34.

4. Weinstein SL, Ponseti IV: Congenital dislocation of the hip. J Bone Joint Surg [Am] 1979, 61:119.

Diagnosis

History

Patients with diabetes mellitus develop foot ulcers with little or no warning. The patients first notice an ulceration when they take off their shoes after a day of often normal activity. They will note blistering, redness, swelling, and sometimes deep ulceration with minimal or no pain. Rarely, the ulcers become infected and the patient will actually present with swelling, redness, fever, and chills with purulent drainage from the ulcer.

Physical findings

Diabetic foot ulcers range in severity from very superficial and clean, without evidence of infection, to a deep wound that penetrates to the bone and is associated with soft tissue or bony infection and soft tissue necrosis. On initial presentation, all diabetic foot ulcers should be classified according to grade and stage, as outlined in the University of Texas Classification System for Diabetic Foot Wounds (Table 1, Fig. 1). Patients with diabetic foot ulcers usually have decreased or no protective sensation. Protective sensation is best tested by using the Semmes-Weinstein monofilament gage system. Perfusion of the limb is frequently impaired in patients with diabetes; an ankle/brachial index measurement of peripheral blood pressure should be obtained to quantify the adequacy of perfusion to the affected lower extremity.

Imaging and laboratory studies

Anterioposterior and lateral radiographs should be obtained for each foot with an ulcer to ensure that the underlying bone is not infected. For patients with impaired perfusion (demonstrated by an ankle/brachial index less than 0.80), more extensive evaluation of the vascular system should be done to assess the adequacy of distal limb perfusion.

Complications

Simple diabetic foot ulcers can cause disastrous complications, resulting in extensive necrosis and deep infection that may lead to amputation of a toe or even amputation of the entire foot if treatment is not aggressive.

Differential diagnosis

Any patient with impaired protective sensation, such as Hansen's disease, can develop an ulcerative lesion of the foot. Sometimes, severe peripheral vascular disease or conditions such as Raynaud's phenomenon lead to skin ulceration in the feet.

Etiology or pathophysiology

Three factors combine to create the diabetic foot ulcer: loss of protective sensation, impaired perfusion, and an impaired immune response. The ulcer starts with an injury that is not perceived or appreciated because of the lack of protective sensation. A simple blister caused by a new pair of shoes will go undetected and unprotected, leading to deep ulceration. Because of impaired perfusion, oxygen and other nutrients and reparative factors are not delivered in sufficient quantity to the injury site and thus cannot initiate or complete the repair process. Because of the impaired immune response, these patients are more susceptible to infection in these open wounds, leading to further tissue necrosis and extension of the infection and creating a limb- or life-threatening situation.

Epidemiology

Almost all patients with diabetes mellitus are susceptible to foot ulcers. They remain one of the most common complications of this disease. The patient's ability to control and heal the ulcers may partly be related to the rigor and aggressiveness of diabetes control. Patients who cannot or do not rigorously control blood glucose levels are more susceptible to diabetic foot ulcers.

Table 1. The University of Texas Classification System for Diabetic Foot Wounds			
	Grade		
Stage	0	1	2	3
A	Pre- or postulcerative lesion completely epithelialized	Superficial wound not involving tendon, capsule, or bone	Wound penetrating to tendon or capsule	Wound penetrating to bone or joint
B	With infection	With infection	With infection	With infection
C	With ischemia	With ischemia	With ischemia	With ischemia
D	With infection and ischemia	With infection and ischemia	With infection and ischemia	With infection and ischemia

From Armstrong et al. [1]; with permission.

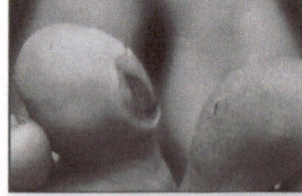

Figure 1. A grade 1, stage A diabetic ulcer of the right great toe.

Treatment

Nonsurgical

Nonsurgical treatment is directed at cleansing and debriding the area of ulceration. Surrounding cellulitis should be treated with appropriate antibiotics. Once a clean, healthy, uninfected ulcer has reached a stable plateau, nonsurgical treatment should be directed at alleviating irritation from weight bearing or shoewear. Otherwise, the ulcer will persist. This goal is often best accomplished using a total-contact cast or pressure-relieving shoe inserts, both of which distribute weight more evenly and alleviate the extensive weight-bearing pressures that cause the persistent or recurrent ulceration. Custom-made shoes with custom-molded innersoles are usually required to prevent recurrent ulcerations and to distribute the weight-bearing forces evenly across the entire foot, in order to minimize the chance of new ulceration.

Surgical

Surgical treatment is reserved for diabetic foot ulcers that do not respond to conservative treatment. Aggressive surgical intervention is sometimes necessary when infection occurs and starts to ascend the affected limb. In these cases, emergency debridement of the necrotic infected focus is mandatory to protect the patient's life and limb. Chronic, recurrent ulcerations may be due to fixed bony deformities that are continuously irritated by weight bearing or shoewear. In these circumstances, the ulcer can be permanently resolved only by removing the underlying, offending bony prominence. Chronic osteomyelitis may develop after repeated, deep ulcerations and may require surgical resection of the infected bone to secure healing of the ulcer.

Exercise and activity modification

Diabetic foot ulcers can be prevented by following some simple rules:

Inspect the feet for skin breakdown and blisters daily.

Wash the feet daily and apply lanolin or baby oil.

Avoid extremes of temperature, especially hot water.

Never put a heating pad or a hot water bottle on either foot.

Do not use chemicals to remove corns and calluses.

Inspect shoes daily for points of irritation.

Wear properly fitting shoes and stockings.

Break in new shoes gradually.

Never walk barefooted.

Treatment aims
To completely heal the ulcer and avoid recurrent ulcerations.

Prognosis
Prognosis directly depends on the severity and depth of the infection. When infection can be eliminated and perfusion of the soft tissues is adequate, healing can be expected. Recurrence of the ulcer, however, is not uncommon.

Follow-up and management
All diabetic patients should be enrolled in a routine foot care program. The program should include the care of toenails, corns, and calluses; repeated instruction about the prevention of ulcerations; and proper foot care techniques.

Key references

1. Armstrong DG, Lavery LA, Harkless LB: Diabetes Care 1998, 21:855–859.

2. Laughlin RT, Calhoun JH, Mader JT: The diabetic foot. J Am Acad Ortho Surg 1995, 3:218–225.

3. Brodsky JW: Outpatient diagnosis and care of the diabetic foot. In Instructional Course Lectures vol 42. Edited by Heckman JD. Rosemont, IL: American Academy of Orthopaedic Surgeons; 1993:121–139.

Diagnosis

History
Difficulty or inability to walk.
Abdominal pain.
Back pain.

Physical findings
Fever is not always present.
Local tenderness may be present.

Imaging and laboratory studies
Radiographs: reveal decreased disk space (Fig. 1). Cases diagnosed late include vertebral body destruction secondary to osteomyelitis.

Bone scan: show increased uptake at adjacent vertebral body or endplate.

Magnetic resonance imaging: findings include increased signal of the disk and either adjacent vertebral body in T2-weighted images. This scan also allows diagnosis of secondary soft tissue inflammatory masses or abscesses (*ie*, psoas abscess).

Laboratory studies: increased leukocyte count, erythrocyte sedimentation rate (ESR), and C-reactive protein level.

Blood cultures: may reveal causative organism.

Aspiration: needle biopsy and culture required if no improvement occurs with treatment.

Complications
Late diagnosis can cause vertebral body destruction and abscess formation requiring surgical drainage. Vertebral destruction can result in scoliosis or kyphosis.

Differential diagnosis
Primary vertebral osteomyelitis.
Septic sacroiliac joint.
Osteoid osteoma.
Scheuerman kyphosis.
Potts disease (tuberculous infection of the spine).

Etiology or pathophysiology
Bacteriologic infection in disk space, probably originating in adjacent vertebral body.
Staphylococcus aureus is the most common organism.
Vascular channels cross the endplate between the vertebral body and disk, allowing infection to cross into the disk and possibly the adjacent vertebra.

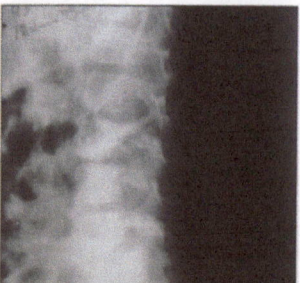

Figure 1. Decreased disk space on lateral radiograph.

Treatment

Nonsurgical

After blood cultures and purified protein derivative testing, antistaphylococci treatment should be initiated. Intravenous antibiotics (first-generation cephalosporin) should be started initially for 3 to 7 days. This is usually sufficient for a dramatic clinical response, with a reduction in the ESR. The next step is oral antibiotics given for 3 to 4 weeks or until the ESR returns to normal.

A thoracic lumbar sacral orthosis or other orthosis may be helpful to relieve symptoms.

Surgical

Surgical drainage with biopsy and culture is necessary for cases that do not respond to conservative care or for those with a soft tissue abscess. Late operative spinal fusion may be needed for the rare cases in which symptoms persist.

Exercise and activity modification

The patient should be able to bear weight with crutches as prescribed by the treating physician.

Treatment aims
To eradicate the infection and eliminate symptoms.

Prognosis
With early recognition and treatment of the condition, prognosis is excellent. Cases diagnosed late may develop osteomyelitis, bone destruction, and deformity.

Follow-up and management
Follow-up radiographs at 6 months are helpful to rule out any late deformity.

Key references

1. Ring D, Johnston CE II, Wenger DR: Pyogenic infectious spondylitis in children: the convergence of diskitis and vertebral osteomyelitis. *J Pediatr Orthop* 1995, 15:652–660.

2. Wenger DR, Bobechko WP, Gilday DO: The spectrum of intervertebral disc-space infection in children. *J Bone Joint Surg* 1978, 60A:100–108.

3. Wenger DR, Davids JR, Ring D: Diskitis and osteomyelitis. In *The Pediatric Spine: Principles and Practice.* Edited by Weinstein SL. New York: Raven Press, 1994:813–835.

Diagnosis

Definition
Dislocation of the hip may occur with or without associated fracture of the acetabulum or the femoral head. Dislocations may also occur in total hip arthroplasties.

History
Bony dislocation is usually due to high-energy trauma, often applied to the affected limb with the hip flexed. Dislocation of total hip arthroplasty can occur with even the most benign movement.

Physical findings
Anterior dislocation (10% to 15% of cases): if anterior/superior, the limb is extended and externally rotated and the head may be palpable anteriorly; if anterior/inferior, the limb is abducted, externally rotated, and flexed.

Posterior dislocation: involved limb is shortened, internally rotated, and adducted.

Imaging and laboratory studies
Radiographs (anteroposterior and lateral) usually demonstrate the gross abnormality. Always include radiographs of the ipsilateral knee to rule out additional fractures.

Computed tomography may be necessary in bony dislocations to assess fractures of the head and the acetabulum.

Complications
Osteonecrosis of the femoral head.

Sciatic nerve damage from posterior dislocation (10% to 14% of cases).

Myositis ossificans.

Posttraumatic arthritis.

Associated femoral shaft fracture.

Differential diagnosis
Femoral neck or intertrochanteric fracture.

Etiology or pathophysiology
Dislocation is caused by severe trauma in the bony hip. Dislocation of a total hip prosthesis may occur because of malposition of the components or excessive range of motion.

Classification
Relationship of head to acetabulum: anterior, posterior, central.
Dislocation with fracture of the head.

Treatment

Nonsurgical
Closed reduction is the treatment of choice unless the acetabulum is unstable or bony fragments become entrapped in the joint. Reduction is done with the Stimson, Allis, or Bigelow maneuvers, each designed to reposition the hip within the joint. Often a combination of maneuvers is necessary.

Surgical
Open reduction may be necessary either in cases of bony fracture or in cases of total hip arthroplasty in which soft tissue becomes interposed within the joint.

Exercise and activity modification
Activity modification must be prescribed for 6 to 8 weeks to allow soft tissues to heal. The patient should be able to bear weight with crutches as prescribed by the treating physician.

Treatment aims
Bony dislocation is an orthopedic emergency, and the hip must be reduced as soon as possible to prevent osteonecrosis of the femoral head.

Prognosis
Risk for osteonecrosis approaches 100% with dislocations that are left out for 24 hours. Reducing the hip within 6 hours of injury greatly reduces the chance of osteonecrosis. Of all patients with posterior fracture-dislocations of the hip, 38% to 48% develop posttraumatic arthritis.

Follow-up and management
Follow-up computed tomography and radiography are necessary in patients with bony dislocation to ensure that no bony fragments are left within the joint. Weight-bearing status is usually touchdown for 2 to 6 weeks. Total hip dislocations are routinely placed in an abduction brace for up to 3 to 6 months to prevent subsequent dislocations.

Key references
1. DeLee JC: Fractures and dislocations of the hip. In *Rockwood and Green's Fractures in Adults.* Edited by Rockwood CA Green DP. Philadelphia: Lippincott–Raven; 1996:1659–1825.

A. Agarwal

Diagnosis

History
Patients with distal humerus fractures present after a traumatic event. This event can be a fall or, more commonly, a motor vehicle collision. Symptoms are pain, swelling, and inability to move the elbow. Patients may also report associated radial, median, or ulnar nerve symptoms. Elderly patients may sustain distal humerus fractures from simple falls; the result may be severely comminuted fractures, often termed a "bag of bones."

Physical findings
The elbow is usually moderately swollen and may be tense. Crepitus is obvious on palpation of the elbow. Motion is difficult to test because of associated gross motion and pain. A thorough neurovascular examination will reveal any associated radial, median, or ulnar nerve symptoms. The radial nerve is most commonly involved. Distal pulses should also be adequately assessed. The associated soft tissue injury must also be assessed because open fractures are surgical emergencies. A significant soft tissue injury can also make surgery much more difficult and may increase the chance of wound complications.

Imaging and laboratory studies
Anteroposterior and lateral radiographs of the affected elbow are the standard diagnostic test (Fig. 1). This will reveal any associated dislocation as well. Because of the mechanism of injury, it is often a good idea to obtain radiographs of both the ipsilateral shoulder and the forearm. If the patient has wrist pain, an antero-posterior and lateral radiograph of the wrist should be taken. For extremely comminuted fractures, computed tomography may help define the anatomy of the fracture. If any vascular compromise is detected, angiography should be done.

Complications
Complications include hardware prominence and the associated olecranon bursitis. This can be painful enough to require removal of the hardware. One of the more common complications is elbow stiffness. Most patients will have some loss of motion and usually of terminal extension. Ulnar neuropathy is a frequent postoperative complication because of the mobilization of the nerve required during reconstructive surgery. The rate of nonunion has been reported to be as high as 15%, but this complication is usually the result of inadequate fixation or nonoperative treatment. There is a high incidence of delayed union or nonunion of olecranon osteotomy performed during the exposure. One third of all complications are related to the osteotomy. Malunion occurs with nonoperative treatment of certain fractures. Posttraumatic arthritis is associated with the comminuted intra-articular fractures. Heterotopic ossification can be a serious complication; if it limits motion, excision may be necessary. Prophylactic measures, such as indomethacin or low-dose radiation, have not been proven effective in any studies, although indomethacin is frequently used. If indomethacin is prescribed, the usual dosage is 25 mg orally three times daily or 75 mg of the slow release form per day. Infection is a rare complication after surgery.

Differential diagnosis
An elbow dislocation or other fractures about the elbow can resemble a fracture of the distal humerus. These injuries include fractures of the radial head, ole-cranon, isolated condyle fractures, capitel-lum, or trochlea. Radiographs help identify the exact abnormality. Occasionally, a sep-tic elbow joint or a neuropathic joint may mimic a fracture.

Etiology or pathophysiology
Distal humerus fractures are caused by a direct mechanical force. The force can hit directly onto the flexed elbow or as an axial load through the forearm on the extended elbow. Low-energy twisting injuries resulting in spiral or distal third fractures also occur, but these are usually related to a pathologic process.

Epidemiology
Distal humerus fractures account for about 1% of adult fractures. Several classi-fication schemes have been devised. One of the most useful classifications is by Müller, who divided the fractures into three types: Type A, nonarticular; Type B, partial articular; Type C, total articular. Within each category, there is an increas-ing degree of severity, designated as 1, 2, and 3. Single fractures of the humeral condyles occur but are less common (less than 5 of all fractures) than true distal humerus fractures.

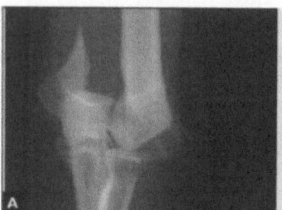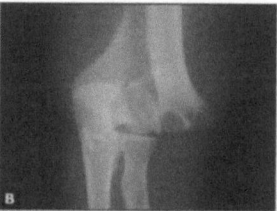

Figure 1. A, Anteroposterior view and B, an attempted lateral view of a distal humerus fracture.

Treatment

Nonsurgical

Some extra-articular fractures can be treated with cast immobilization after closed reduction. Splint or cast immobilization is used initially for 2 to 3 weeks. This is followed by use of a hinged functional brace with early range of motion. Olecranon traction is occasionally used but is not ideal. If patient factors contraindicate surgical treatment, nonsurgical treatment prevails.

Surgical

Open reduction with internal fixation (ORIF) is the best way to manage distal humerus fractures that involve the articular surface. Even some Type A fractures should be managed with ORIF, although some can be treated without surgery. Many factors must be considered before surgery is chosen for a distal humerus fracture. These factors include the patient's age, quality of bone, soft tissue status, and fracture anatomy or presence of comminution. Open fractures require emergency irrigation and debridement, with stabilization if the soft tissue allows. External fixation may be used until the soft tissue envelope is amenable to ORIF. Several exposures can be used to perform ORIF. For fractures that involve both the medial and lateral columns, the posterior approach with an olecranon osteotomy (articular fractures) or without an osteotomy (extra-articular fractures) should be used. The medial or lateral approaches are best for single-column involvement. Olecranon osteotomies can be performed extra-articularly or intra-articularly. They should be predrilled for placement of a 6.5-mm cancellous screw. Fixation of the fracture itself is dictated by the fracture pattern, and preoperative planning as described by the AO/ASIF group is extremely helpful. A combination of lag screws and plate fixation is the best method. Plates can be 3.5-mm pelvic reconstruction, 3.5-mm dynamic compression, or one third tubular plates. The reconstruction plate and the dynamic compression plate are the best implants. Specialized plates can also be used. In general, bicolumnar fixation should be performed with two plates (in addition to lag screw fixation) placed 90° to each other if possible (Fig. 2). One is placed medially, and the other is placed posteriorly on the lateral column. This has been shown to be the most stable construct. If significant bone loss accompanies the injury, bone grafting may be needed, either at the initial surgery to help reconstruct the anatomy or later on to expedite healing.

Exercise and activity modification

Exercise and activity modifications are dictated by the treatment. As a general rule, no heavy lifting is allowed during rehabilitation. Gentle active and active-assist motion is allowed. The use of passive motion is somewhat controversial because it has been linked to heterotopic ossification. Activities of daily living can be performed after the initial period of immobilization.

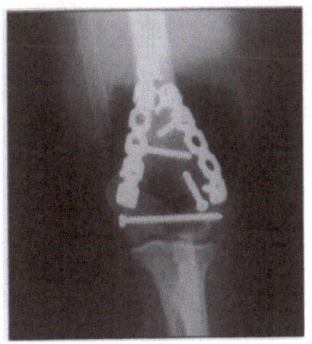

Figure 2. The results of open reduction and internal fixation through a posterior approach with an olecranon osteotomy.

Key references

1. Helfet DL, Schmeling GJ: Bicondylar intraarticular fractures of the distal humerus in adults. Clin Orthop 1993, 292:26–36.

2. Ring DR, Jupiter JB: Complex fractures of the distal humerus and their complications. J Shoulder Elbow Surg 1999, 8:85–97.

3. Scemitsch EH, Tencer AF, Henley MB: Biomechanical evaluation of methods of internal fixation of the distal humerus. J Orthop Trauma 1994, 8:468–475.

4. Webb LX: Distal humerus fractures in adults. J Am Acad Orthop Surg 1996, 4:336–344.

Diagnosis

History
Fall on an outstretched arm.
Localized pain over the distal forearm.

Physical findings
Swelling, tenderness, and possible deformity at the fracture site.
Neurologic examination should always be performed.

Imaging and laboratory studies
Radiographs: anteroposterior and lateral radiograph of the forearm should include the joint above and below the injury (other ipsilateral fractures are not uncommon and are often missed).

Complications
Compartment syndrome or carpal tunnel syndrome.
Injury to the median nerve caused by displaced fractures.
Growth disturbance rarely occurring in physeal injuries of the distal radius.
Malunion of the fracture.
Reflex sympathetic dystrophy.

Differential diagnosis
Contusion.
Wrist sprain.
Carpal fracture and dislocation.

Etiology or pathophysiology
Indirect mechanism is most common, secondary to a fall on an outstretched arm.
Direct trauma.

Epidemiology
Most common fracture in the immature skeleton.
Male predominance is 3:1.

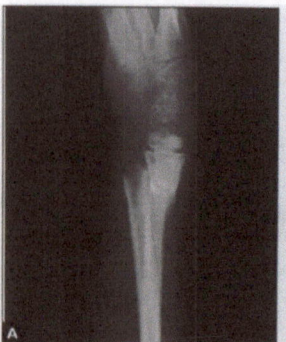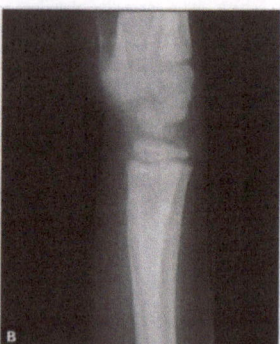

Figure 1. Distal radius fracture (A) in a boy aged 8 years that spontaneously remodeled (B).

Treatment

Nonsurgical

Torus fractures and nondisplaced distal radius fractures must be immobilized for about 4 weeks in a splint or cast. The need to reduce displaced distal radial fractures, either physeal or metaphyseal, depends on the displacement, clinical presentation, and age of the patient. For physeal fractures, up to 50% apposition and less than 25° of angulation can be accepted if at least 1 year of growth remains. Angulated metaphyseal fractures are reduced if the deformity is cosmetically obvious (usually greater than 15° or 20°). The need to reduce an apex dorsal deformity is greater because of the poor cosmetic appearance and tendency to lose supination with these fractures. Bayonet fractures are usually reduced, although bayonet apposition will remodel if 3 years of growth remain (Fig. 1). Fracture reduction is usually accomplished with conscious sedation and regional anesthesia.

After fracture reduction, short arm casts or long arm casts that are univalved should maintain the reduction if there is a good three-point mold. Sugartong splints are acceptable. Four weeks of immobilization is needed for physeal fractures, and up to 8 weeks is needed for metaphyseal fractures.

Surgical

Closed reduction and percutaneous pinning are required if an acceptable reduction cannot be maintained with a cast or in the presence of ipsilateral fractures. Open reduction with internal fixation is necessary when an acceptable reduction cannot be achieved by closed methods or when open fractures must be debrided. A single, small-diameter bicortical pin (0.062 in) inserted through the radial styloid for physeal fractures or inserted just proximal to the physis for metaphyseal fractures is usually sufficient. At 3 weeks, the fracture has usually become sufficiently stable to allow removal of the pin. All fractures into the distal articular surface should be anatomically reduced and stabilized.

Treatment aims
To obtain and maintain an acceptable reduction with no significant residual deformity or decreased function.

Prognosis
Most of these fractures are treated successfully by closed methods.

Follow-up and management
Weight-dependent dosages of oral narcotics are necessary for children because higher dosages can mask the onset of a compartment syndrome. Previously manipulated or unstable fractures should be checked at 2 weeks to make sure alignment has not changed. Univalved casts may be overwrapped at that time. For physeal fractures, follow-up radiographs are often obtained 4 to 6 months after injury to rule out growth disturbance.

Key references
1. Wilkins KE, O'Brien ET: Fractures of the distal radius and ulna. In *Fractures in Children*. Edited by Rockwood CA, Wilkins KE, Beaty JH. Philadelphia: Lippincott–Raven; 1996:451–515.

Diagnosis

Physical findings

Painless nodules in the palm of the hand with progressive contracture of the finger. The progress of the contracture and the extent of the contracture vary substantially. Pads may form over the dorsum of the proximal interphalangeal joint.

May be associated with fascial nodules in the foot (Fig. 1) along the plantar surface and nodular bands in the penis (Peyronie's disease).

There are familial variations, and association with diabetes, epilepsy, and liver disease has been reported.

Imaging and laboratory studies

Medical work-up should include studies to rule out diabetes and liver disease.

Differential diagnosis

Contractures with no palmar fascial component can occur from trauma or congenital variants.
Palmar fibrosis with no contracture can occur in patients with diabetes.

Etiology or pathophysiology

No specific causative agent, but there are definite familial tendencies.
Essential feature is development of fibroblasts and thickening in the palmar fascia.
Early onset before age 40 usually produces rapid contractures and recurrence.
Knuckle pads.
Peyronie's disease.
Fascial thickening in sole of foot.
Epilepsy.
Liver disease.

Epidemiology

Contractures usually begin in patients in their late 40s, and are seen more often in men of European descent.
Rare in Asians and Africans.

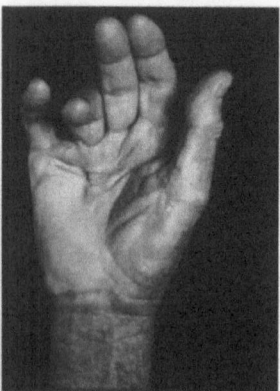

Figure 1. Dupuytren's contracture involves the palmar fascia and can result in nodules in the hand and a fixed flexion contracture of any of the digits of the hand. As shown in this case involving the ring finger, the central cord proximal to the base of the metacarpophalangeal joint results in flexion contractures of both the metacarpophalangeal joint and the proximal interphalangeal joint.

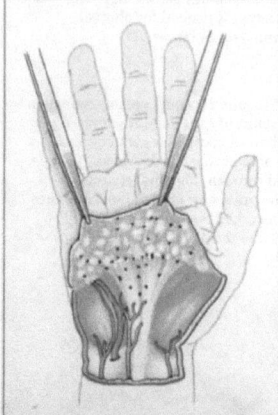

Figure 2. The pathologic process involved in Dupuytren's contracture is the result of nodules and cord formation in the palmar fascia, which produces the contractures in the digits. Portions of the skin and the subcutaneous tissue also may need to be resected when treating Dupuytren's contracture.

F.G. Corley **DUPUYTREN'S CONTRACTURE**

Treatment

Nonsurgical
No lasting benefits have been seen with nonsurgical treatment.

Surgical
Surgical management is directed toward preventing and relieving contractures through partially or totally removing the palmar fascia (Fig. 2). Metacarpophalangeal joint contractures are more easily relieved than are proximal interphalangeal joint contractures.

Treatment aims
To release contracture and prevent proximal interphalangeal joint contracture.

Prognosis
Depends on the severity of the contracture, the age of the patient, and the incidence of postoperative complications. Proximal interphalangeal joint contractures are significantly more difficult to correct than metacarpophalangeal joint contractures. A younger age at onset usually results in more severe contractures and the possibility of recurrence.

Follow-up and management
Postoperative splinting and occupational therapy are usually routine for contractures. Complications include digital nerve and artery injury, skin loss, infection, stiffness, and reflex dystrophy.

Key references
1. Benson LS, Williams CS, Kable M: Dupuytren's contracture. J Am Acad Orthop Surg 1998, 6:24–35.
2. Schneider LH, Hankin FM, Eisenberg T: Surgery of Dupuytren's disease: a review of the open palm method. J Hand Surg 1986, 11A:23–27.
3. Seyfer AE, Hueston JT: Dupuytren's contracture. Hand Clin 1991, 7:46.
4. Strickland JW, Leibovic SJ: Anatomy and pathogenesis of the digital cords and nodules. Hand Clin 1991, 7:645–657.

Diagnosis

History

The most common cause of elbow dislocation is a fall on an outstretched hand with the elbow in extension and abduction. If the force is great, the skin in the cubital fossa can be torn, resulting in an open dislocation.

Physical findings

If the patient is examined shortly after injury, the findings are fairly typical. The forearm appears shortened, and the cubital fossa appears full. The olecranon process is easily palpable posteriorly. Often the skin just proximal to the olecranon is puckered and redundant. Late presentation of the injury reveals an extremity with diffuse swelling around the elbow. A careful neurovascular examination should be performed before reduction of the dislocation is attempted.

Imaging and laboratory studies

Routine orthogonal radiographs should allow classification of the dislocation (Fig. 1).

Complications

Vascular and nerve injury can occur at the time of the dislocation. After relocation of the elbow, ligament calcification and heterotopic ossification can develop in the periarticular soft tissue, causing loss of elbow motion or ankylosis. Unlike with the shoulder, recurrent elbow dislocation is rare.

Differential diagnosis

A pure elbow dislocation must be differentiated from a fracture or fracture-dislocation about the elbow. The more common fractures in this region include those of the extra-articular and intra-articular distal humerus, radial head, and olecranon. The main fracture-dislocations are an elbow dislocation with fracture of the medial humeral epicondyle and an ulna fracture with dislocation of the radial head at the radiocapitellar articulation (a Monteggia injury).

Etiology or pathophysiology

With longitudinal force applied distal to the elbow, the elbow becomes extended. The tip of the olecranon contacts the osseous roof of the distal humeral olecranon fossa and becomes a hinge that rotates posteriorly out of the elbow joint. As this occurs, tensile forces anterior to the elbow cause capsular rupture and brachialis muscle injury. Associated forearm pronation or supination with elbow hyperextension may cause posterolateral or posteromedial dislocation of the proximal radius and ulna.

Epidemiology

The most common type of dislocation is posterior. Pure posterior dislocations are less common than posterolateral. Other uncommon types include medial, anterior, lateral, and divergent dislocations.

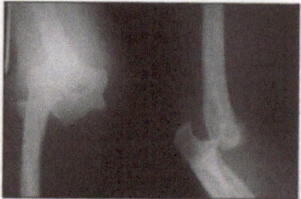

Figure 1. Two views of a dislocated elbow.

Treatment

Nonsurgical
Most elbow dislocations should be treated with a single gentle, closed relocation. Before any manipulation of the upper extremity, a careful neurovascular evaluation of the extremity should be performed. After relocation, this examination should be repeated and the elbow passively moved to determine the limit of elbow stability. Mechanical blocks to motion are also sought. Relocation maneuvers have been described with the patient either supine or prone. Analgesia and muscle relaxation are important factors for facilitating a gentle relocation.

Surgical
If forceful attempts at a closed reduction of the elbow have been unsuccessful, an open reduction should be performed. The joint should be explored and injury debris removed. This debris includes blood, articular cartilage, and small osteochondral fractures. The ulnar and radial collateral ligaments should be identified and repaired if torn. If vascular compromise occurs at the time of injury or with closed elbow relocation, vascular exploration of the brachial artery is imperative.

Treatment aims
To achieve full, active elbow motion with no recurrence of dislocation or subluxation.

Prognosis
The prognosis for a closed dislocation is generally very good. Many patients will lose a few degrees of active elbow extension, but this is rarely of functional significance. The rate of recurrence of dislocation is low.

Follow-up and management
After the elbow has been relocated, orthogonal radiographs should be taken to verify that the elbow is in place. Immobilization of the elbow in at least 90° of flexion is generally used to maintain the relocation. Controversy exists over the recommended period of elbow immobilization before active motion is begun, ranging from 1 day to 3 weeks. Periodic follow-up is important to determine that active motion is returning to normal. If the return of motion is slowed or halted, passive extension with an orthosis may be necessary to improve motion without surgery. Surgical release of the joint and surrounding soft tissue may be required if orthotic treatment fails. Chronic recurrence of the dislocation necessitates surgical reconstruction of the joint.

Key references
1. Linscheid RL, Wheeler DK: Elbow dislocations. JAMA 1965, 194:1171–1176.
2. Josefsson PO, Gentz CF, Johnell O, Wendeberg B: Surgical versus non-surgical treatment of ligamentous injuries following dislocation of the elbow joint: a prospective randomized study. J Bone Joint Surg 1987, 69A:605–608.
3. O'Driscoll S: Elbow instability. Hand Clin 1994, 10:405–415.

Diagnosis

History

Patients report pain in the elbow and forearm area that is localized to the medial or, more commonly, the lateral side of the elbow. It is often described as a burning pain that emanates from the elbow region into the forearm. Onset of pain is insidious, and its occurrence is associated with use. Sports or performance of job activities may exacerbate symptoms.

Physical findings

Palpation around the elbow reveals tenderness over the lateral or medial epicondyle. Tenderness is present over the extensor region if the symptoms are lateral and if over the flexor-pronator origin the symptoms are medial. In patients with lateral epicondylitis, pain is exacerbated with resistance to wrist extension and long finger extension while the elbow is held in extension. Conversely, pain in medial epicondylitis worsens with resistance to wrist flexion and forearm pronation with the elbow in extension. Neurologic deficits are usually absent, although mild weakness may be present. Concomitant ulnar neuropathy can occur with medial-sided pain. Minimal to no swelling occurs. Diagnosis is made by history and the above findings.

Imaging and laboratory studies

No laboratory studies are indicated, although a complete blood count and erythrocyte sedimentation rate can be done to rule out other diseases. Similarly, plain radiographs are negative and are used more to rule out bony abnormality. A small percentage of patients may exhibit calcification in the soft tissues. Cervical spine radiographs may be needed to rule out spine problems.

Complications

Chronic pain is the most common problem associated with epicondylitis. However, most complications are primarily related to the surgical treatment of this condition. Transient ulnar paresthesias and failure to relieve pain are the two most common complications.

Differential diagnosis

Any condition around the elbow can be confused with epicondylitis, including fractures, dislocations, tendonitis, and tumors. Radial tunnel syndrome, in which the posterior interosseous nerve is compressed, can be differentiated from lateral epicondylitis by exacerbation of pain with resistance to middle finger extension or forearm supination with the elbow extended. Differentiation can be difficult because both are associated with pain at the lateral epicondyle. Electromyography may reveal abnormalities in the radial nerve with radial tunnel syndrome. Osteochondral defects of the elbow can also result in a similar picture. Another part of the differential diagnosis is cervical spine disease with radiculopathy.

Etiology or pathophysiology

Epicondylitis, an overuse syndrome, occurs from an indirect injury caused by repetitious activities. Affected patients have repetitive tension overload in both the forearm and wrist extensors. Pathologic studies showed degenerative tears in the extensor or flexor origins. A direct tear has been shown in only 10% to 20% of cases. Cellular proliferation and microscopic abnormalities of the extensor carpi radialis brevis muscle are consistent with a degenerative process rather than an inflammatory process. The pronator teres and flexor carpi radialis are most commonly involved in medial epicondylitis. Recurrent valgus forces to the elbow contribute to the development of medial-sided abnormality.

Epidemiology

Epicondylitis is classified as medial or lateral. Lateral epicondylitis is commonly known as "tennis elbow." It is the most common clinical dysfunction of the elbow, making up 85% to 95% of all cases. Approximately 10% to 50% of all tennis players develop this condition. The peak incidence occurs between the fourth and fifth decades of life, and there is a slight male predominance. Tennis players older than 40 years of age have an increased risk. The dominant arm is affected three times as often as the nondominant arm. Medial epicondylitis, which accounts for 10% to 15% of cases, is called "golfer's elbow," although baseball pitchers are also prone to develop it.

Treatment

Nonsurgical

Nonsurgical treatment is the mainstay of current therapy. Treatment should consist of rest, anti-inflammatory medications, ice, stretching, and strengthening exercises. Phonophoresis can be added, and forearm bands that help to relieve the tension can be used. Patient education is also an important component of treatment. Patients must be counseled about lifestyle modifications that may help alleviate pain. Steroid injections into the muscle origin can help. Conservative therapy should be tried for at least 3 months before surgical intervention is attempted. Most cases will resolve with an appropriate treatment plan.

Surgical

Surgical intervention is rarely indicated because most cases resolve with nonoperative management. Approximately 5% to 10% of cases become recalcitrant and may require surgery. There are four basic procedural options for lateral epicondylitis: 1) relieving the tension in the tendon, 2) repairing the degenerative tendon, 3) denervating radial nerve, and 4) using intra-articular procedures. Surgical release of the tendon and lengthening procedures are common ways to relieve the tension. These can, however, cause residual weakness. Fewer options are available for medial-sided abnormalities. The most popular is resection of the degenerative tissue and reapproximation of the tendon. Release-type procedures done medially result in unacceptable weakness.

Exercise and activity modification

These aspects become an important component in the treatment of any overuse disorder. Rest is of paramount importance to help relieve symptoms. Sports must be restricted in the initial phase, and sporting activity techniques may then have to be altered. An analysis of the patient's motions can reveal the cause of the abnormality. For example, if the patient's backhand stroke in tennis is the problem, this stroke can be adjusted. Additional changes in the workplace may help alleviate symptoms.

Treatment aims
The goal of treatment is pain relief. Once pain is alleviated, patients can return to work or the activities they enjoy.

Prognosis
Most patients respond to nonoperative measures. More than 80% of patients with chronic lateral cases will obtain good relief with surgery. Good or excellent results can be obtained in 95% of patients undergoing surgical treatment of medial epicondylitis.

Follow-up and management
In the initial acute phase, the elbow may be splinted for 2 weeks. After this, active elbow exercises can be started. A program of elbow strengthening should begin at 4 weeks, with resistive flexion or extension exercises commencing at 6 weeks. A forearm band can also be used initially. Steroid injections, if used, should be given at 3-month intervals at the most. These have provided relief in up to 90% of patients. Unfortunately, pain will recur in as many as 50% of those patients. At the end of 2 months, most patients should have regained adequate strength in the forearm musculature. Use of the forearm band can be continued for several months thereafter. If symptoms continue after 6 to 12 months, surgical intervention should be considered.

Key references
1. Gabel GT, Morrey BF: Tennis elbow. In *Instructional Course Lectures* vol 47. Edited by Cannon WD Jr. Rosemont, IL: American Academy of Orthopaedic Surgeons. 1998:165–172.
2. Jobe FW, Ciccotti MG: Lateral and medial epicondylitis of the elbow. *J Am Acad Orthop Surg* 1994, 2:1–8.

Diagnosis

History

Patellar tendon ruptures occur in athletically active individuals, especially athletes in their third or fourth decade who are involved in jumping sports such as basketball. The injury usually occurs when the athlete lands from a jump and the extensor mechanism is overpowered by the deceleration force created by landing. The athlete usually falls, with immediate pain and swelling and difficulty walking. Patients frequently note prodromal symptoms of anterior knee pain as a result of patellar tendinitis.

Physical findings

Immediately after injury, swelling and tenderness in the area of the patellar tendon occur. On palpation, a defect that is usually directly distal to the patella can be felt. The patient cannot perform a straight-leg raise and notes pain in the area of the patellar tendon. The patella may be "high riding" or in a more proximal position than the contralateral normal knee (patella alta) (Fig. 1).

Imaging and laboratory studies

Radiographs should be obtained for evaluation of patellar fractures, avulsion fragments, and the presence of a proximally positioned ("high riding") patella. Magnetic resonance imaging is diagnostic of such an injury, but physical examination and plain radiography are usually adequate for establishing a correct diagnosis.

Complications

Failure to diagnose an acute patellar tendon rupture will lead to chronic disability, extension weakness, and quadriceps scarring. The gap secondary to the injury will not close because of the viscoelasticity and proximal migration of the extensor mechanism.

Differential diagnosis

An acute flexion force to the knee, such as from a fall or landing after a jump, can also cause a quadriceps tendon rupture. This injury also produces anterior knee pain, swelling, soft tissue gap, or defect, but these occur superior to the patellar tendon. Patients with a quadriceps tendon rupture are also unable to actively extend the knee. The location of a defect above (quadriceps tendon rupture) or below (patellar tendon rupture) the patella determines the location of injury. Patellar fractures can be caused by a flexion injury but usually result from a fall with a direct blow to the anterior knee. Radiographs are necessary to rule out a fracture of the patella.

Etiology or pathophysiology

Middle-aged adults are prone to patellar tendon or quadriceps tendon rupture. The insertion of the quadriceps and patellar tendon as the patella undergoes tendinosis or degenerative changes weakens the insertion of the tendon fibers. Patellar tendon ruptures occur most commonly in patients under 40 years of age; quadriceps tears occur in patients over 40 years of age.

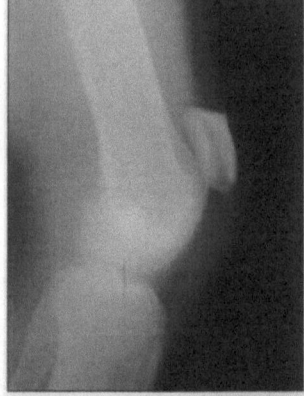

Figure 1. Radiograph of a patellar tendon rupture.

Treatment

Nonsurgical

Only extremely debilitated or medically compromised patients should be treated nonsurgically. Such treatment does not allow for approximation of tendon ends and does not prevent muscle shortening and leg weakness.

Surgical

A ruptured patellar tendon is repaired surgically with direct exposure of the torn ends. The patellar tendon usually avulses from the patella and is reattached with heavy nonabsorbable braided sutures through drill holes in the patella. Patellar tendon repairs can be protected with a figure eight tension band construct that extends from the superior edge of the patella distal to the tibial tubercle. This allows protection during range-of-motion exercises. Early weight bearing is allowed in a brace or knee immobilizer. If a wire figure eight tension band is not used, immobilization for 3 weeks in extension is recommended to protect the repair. Recent studies have evaluated early range of motion with primary repair of the patellar tendon and without augmentation. Quadriceps tendon rupture is repaired in a similar fashion depending on the type of tear. No wire construct exists to protect a quadriceps repair; thus, short-term immobilization in extension is used.

Exercise and activity modification

No preventive measures are available. Patients with patellar tendinitis are at greater risk for rupture with continued high-intensity jumping activities. Decreasing jumping activities may help prevent injury.

Treatment aims

To restore the integrity of the patellar tendon and restore the normal musculotendinous length of the quadriceps. Healing in a lengthened position with quadriceps scarring will result in chronic weakness, limp, and inability to perform jumping activities.

Prognosis

With prompt repair, the prognosis for return to function is excellent. Delay in diagnosis frequently leads to quadriceps muscle contracture and difficult reconstructive options. Patellar tendon ruptures that are brought to medical attention late are usually reconstructed with transfer of the semitendinosus and gracilis tendons through the patella.

Follow-up and management

With wire protection, early range of motion can be instituted. Healing usually takes place 6 to 9 weeks after injury, and patients should wait 4 to 6 months after injury to return to sports.

Key references

1. Kelly DW, Carter VS, Jobe FW, et al.: Patella and quadriceps tendon ruptures: jumpers' knee. *Am J Sports Med* 1984, 12:375–380.

2. Marder RA, Timmerman LA: Primary repair of patellar tendon rupture without augmentation. *Am J Sports Med* 1999, 3:304–309.

Diagnosis

History

Femoral shaft fractures are usually the result of high-energy injuries. Most patients are involved in motor vehicle collisions or motorcycle accidents or are pedestrians hit by automobiles. Other mechanisms can be responsible, such as falls from heights or gunshot wounds. In elderly patients who sustain femur fractures, the fractures are often the result of low-energy force and are caused by pathologic bone due to osteoporosis or tumors (commonly metastatic). When young patients sustain femur fractures with a trivial injury, one must suspect a pathologic process such as a tumor.

Physical findings

Patients present with pain, deformity, shortening, swelling, and inability to bear weight on the affected extremity. Gross motion and crepitus are noted on palpation of the thigh. Associated open soft tissue injuries may or may not be present. If a laceration or open wound is present, the fracture should be considered open until proven otherwise. The thigh can swell extensively because of blood loss; the average blood loss has been reported to be as high as 1200 mL. However, thigh compartment syndrome is rare. Almost as important as evaluation of the injured extremity is assessment for associated injuries. It is crucial to assess for ipsilateral hip (acetabulum, intertrochanteric, femoral neck), knee (distal femur, tibial plateau, tibia, ankle, and foot injuries. It is also important to check for other organ system injuries.

Imaging and laboratory studies

Radiographs should be obtained promptly. Anteroposterior and lateral femur films are the standard (Fig. 1). One must also evaluate the ipsilateral knee and hip with radiographs. Depending on the amount of comminution involved, assessing radiographs of the contralateral femur with a measuring stick can help judge the length of nail needed. Computed tomography can be considered if a pathologic fracture is suspected. Magnetic resonance imaging is rarely if ever indicated.

Complications

Failure to diagnose a femur fracture secondary to a pathologic process, especially in the young patient with a primary tumor, can be disastrous. Nonunion is an uncommon problem with modern operative techniques and occurs less than 2% of the time. Delayed union is a problem but is more common with open and higher-energy injuries, which have a significant soft tissue component. Pudendal nerve palsy secondary to fracture table use has been described. Malunion can occur with valgus or varus angulation. Rotational malalignment (7% of cases) can also be a significant problem. Leg length discrepancy occurs about 2% of the time. An associated vascular injury may develop (eg, femoral artery at adductor hiatus) and can be limb- or life-threatening. Another complication is failure of the implant, which is primarily due to fatigue failure. Rare complications include infection (1% of cases), nerve injury, and compartment syndrome. Heterotopic ossification about the hip, which is clinically significant, occurs in less than 5% of the patients treated with antegrade nailing. Acute respiratory distress syndrome has been noted in approximately 2% of patients treated with reamed intramedullary nailing.

Differential diagnosis

The diagnosis of an acute femur fracture is usually very clear. Gross instability of the thigh can be mimicked by a hip or knee dislocation. The level of fracture of the femur can vary, and the fracture may not affect the shaft but rather may be located very distally or proximally; thus, the treatment decisions would be much different.

Etiology or pathophysiology

Femoral shaft fractures are caused by direct mechanical force. The typical scenario is dashboard-to-knee injury. Another mechanism is more direct, such as a motor vehicle–pedestrian accident.

Epidemiology

Rate of injury is 1 to 3 cases per 10,000 people. Most patients are young, especially in the third or fourth decades of life, although the age varies widely. Injuries tend to occur in a bimodal distribution, either in persons younger than 25 years of age or those older than 65 years of age. The elderly population often has low-energy injuries that may be pathologic in origin.

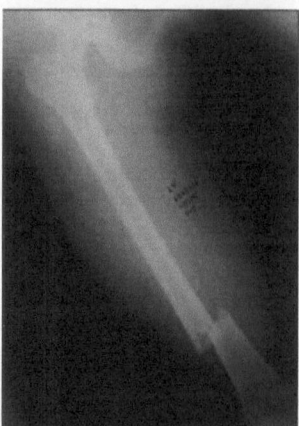

Figure 1. Anteroposterior view of a right distal-third to mid-third junction femoral shaft fracture.

Treatment

Nonsurgical

Skeletal Traction: this method was once used for definitive treatment but today is used for temporary and early fracture care before surgery. It can be used as an adjunct intraoperatively, either on the fracture table or regular bed, to help with reduction of the fracture. Occasionally, it is used for patients too sick to undergo surgery, but this is a poor alternative.

Cast Brace: this method is used after an initial trial of skeletal traction. It allows progressive weight bearing once the fracture has somewhat consolidated in traction, but it is rarely used.

Surgical

Intramedullary Nails: the antegrade technique with reaming is the gold standard for most femoral shaft fractures. All nails are usually statically locked. Retrograde intramedullary nailing is becoming more popular. It has results similar to those seen with the antegrade procedure, and has no long-term adverse effects on the knee joint. The technique is useful for patients with multiple injuries; those with bilateral femur fractures; and those with ipsilateral acetabular, pelvic, or femoral neck fractures. It is also useful for patients with a "floating knee" injury (ie, ipsilateral tibia fracture).

Open Reduction and Internal Fixation: this technique is occasionally used. It requires extensive dissection of fracture through a lateral approach and compression plating of fracture with broad 4.5 dynamic compression plate. This technique can sometimes be useful when an associated vascular injury requires repair.

External Fixation: this is an acceptable alternative for patients with severe open soft tissue injuries. It is also useful in the unstable patient as a quick technique to stabilize the femur fracture.

Exercise and activity modification

During the healing period, the patient requires extensive rehabilitation exercises to help maintain the strength of the leg and range of motion of the hip and knee joints. Quad sets, short arc quads, straight-leg raises, and isometric exercises are useful in maintaining quadriceps strength. Range of motion of the hip and, especially, the knee can be active, active-assist, and passive. Knee effusion, present in most patients, subsides in 2 to 6 weeks and may initially limit motion. Athletes with femur fractures may require hardware removal (intramedullary nail or plate) before returning to contact sports, although this area is controversial.

Treatment aims

Surgical: To stabilize femur, allow early mobilization of the patient, and to maintain proper alignment of femur during healing process.
Nonsurgical: To stabilize femur, and restore and maintain femoral length, angulation, and rotation until definitive fracture care can be performed.

Prognosis

Prognosis depends on many factors, such as the degree of comminution, nature of injury (open vs closed), and associated injuries. Overall, prognosis with healing of fracture is excellent; usual healing time is 14 to 18 weeks. In 95% of patients, normal hip and knee motion will return. Infection rates are extremely low.

Follow-up and management

Immediate mobilization can occur after stabilization of femur. Weight-bearing depends on the method of fracture fixation and degree of comminution. For intramedullary nails immediate partial weight bearing can be used for Winquist 0 and I fractures. Patients with Winquist II and III fractures can begin with toe-touch weight bearing and progress to partial weight bearing in 4 to 6 weeks as the fracture consolidates. Winquist IV fractures may require prolonged toe-touch weight bearing until abundant fracture callous is evident. For open reduction with internal and external fixation patients usually require prolonged toe-touch weight-bearing until healing. Follow-up should continue until the fracture heals and for at least 1 year thereafter.

Key references

1. Brumback RJ, Ellison TS, Poka A, et al.: Intramedullary nailing of femoral shaft fractures: Part III. Long term effects of static interlocking fixation. J Bone Joint Surg 1992, 74A:106–112.

2. Bucholz RW, Brumback RJ: Fractures of the shaft of the femur. In Rockwood and Green's Fractures in Adults. Edited by Rockwood CA, Green DP, Bucholz RW, et al. Philadelphia: Lippincott–Raven; 1996:1827–1918.

3. Ostrum RF: Treatment of femoral shaft fractures with intramedullary interlocking nails. Am J Orthop 1996, 25(suppl): 4–8.

Diagnosis

History
Gradual onset of pain after puncture wound or injury.

Physical findings
Pain.
Paresthesia.
Swelling.
Erythema (Fig. 1).
Tenderness.
Pain with movement.
Drainage.
Vesicle formation.
Erythema.
Flexion of distal interphalangeal joint.

Imaging and laboratory studies
Radiography may show bone involvement; possible foreign body.
Complete blood count shows elevated leukocyte count.

Complications
Osteomyelitis of distal phalanx.
Loss of pulp of fingertip.
Flexor tenosynovitis.
Loss of fingertip.

Differential diagnosis
Herpetic whitlow—usually has clear vesicles.
Cellulitis of fingertip.
Metastatic tumor.
Calcific tendonitis.

Etiology or pathophysiology
Idiopathic.
Fracture wound.
Bacteria seeding a hematoma.
Fever.
Leukocytosis.
Seen in diabetic patients and immunosuppressed patients.
The septa of the fingertip are involved in the process and can be destroyed, causing a dysfunctional fingertip (Fig. 2).

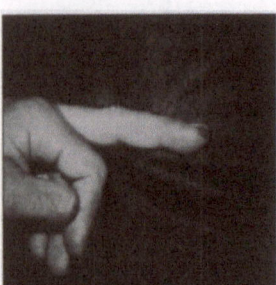

Figure 1. A felon is an infection involving the fingertip. The signs and symptoms—pain, swelling, erythema, and tenderness at the fingertip—are usually preceded by a puncture wound.

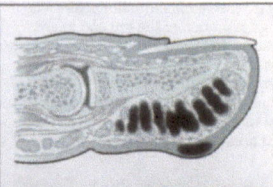

Figure 2. The fingertip is a specialized structure with septa radiating from the distal phalanx to the skin. These septa give support to the fat pad of the distal phalanx. To treat an infection of the distal phalanx or a felon the septa must be surgically divided in order to evacuate the purulent material contained in this closed space infection.

Treatment

Nonsurgical

Nonsurgical treatment should be considered in all injuries. Elevation, splinting, and broad-spectrum antibiotics may be of benefit early on and may negate the need for surgery.

Tetanus prophylaxis.

Surgical

Most felons (Fig. 1) with abscess formation require surgical drainage under aseptic technique, regional anesthesia, and antibiotics.

Treatment aims
To prevent necrosis of fingertip and osteomyelitis of distal phalanx.

Prognosis
Usually good with proper treatment, even for patients with osteomyelitis. Diabetic and immunosuppressed patients present a difficult problem.

Follow-up and management
After surgery and 24 hours of intravenous antibiotics, soaks and oral antibiotic therapy can be started.
Wound is left open and followed for 3 to 5 days initially; thereafter, wound should be monitored weekly.

Key references

1. Abrams RA, Botte MJ: Hand infections: treatment recommendations for specific types. *J Am Acad Orthop Surg* 1996, 4:219–230.

2. Bednar MS, Lane LB: Eponychial marsupialization and nail removal for surgical treatment of chronic paronychia. *J Hand Surg* 1991, 16A:314–317.

3. Bisno AL, Stevens DL: Streptococcal infections of skin and soft tissues. *N Engl J Med* 1996, 240:245.

4. Clarke HJ, Jinnah RH, Byank RP, et al.: *Clostridium difficile* infection in orthopaedic patients. *J Bone Joint Surg* 1990, 72A:1056–1059.

5. Kozin SH, Bishop AT: Atypical mycobacterium infections of the upper extremity. *J Hand Surg* 1994, 19A:480–487.

Diagnosis

History

Occasionally, a child may report vague aching in the plantar aspect of the midfoot with activity.

Physical findings

Loss of normal longitudinal arch in stance (Fig. 1). An arch is present, however, during non–weight-bearing or standing on tiptoe.

With hindfoot valgus, a tight heel cord may be present.

Imaging and laboratory studies

Weight-bearing radiographs: usually unnecessary. Loss of the arch is associated with plantarflexion of the talus. Whereas the axis of the talus and first metatarsal normally line up, increasing flatfoot deformity is associated with an increasing angulation or sag between these lines (Fig. 2).

Computed tomography of the foot: useful only to confirm a possible tarsal coalition (rigid flatfoot).

Complications

Occasional difficulty with shoewear.

Differential diagnosis

Tarsal coalition
Presents with rigid flatfoot in an adolescent or teenager.

Neuromuscular disease (ie, cerebral palsy).

Vertical talus
Presents with rigid flatfoot in a newborn.

Etiology or pathophysiology
Excessive ligamentous laxity is believed to cause flexible flatfoot deformity. Any bony changes are secondary.

Epidemiology
Affects 10% to 20% of the population.

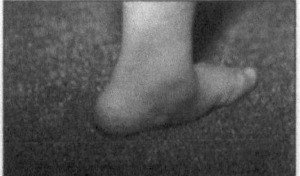

Figure 1. Clinical presentation of flatfoot deformity.

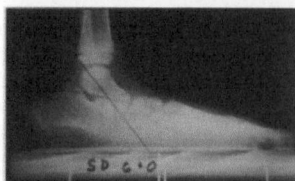

Figure 2. Angulation between the axis of the talus and first ray.

Treatment

Nonsurgical

Heelcord stretching is first step in treating symptomatic patients. Patients with tight heelcords will not respond to other conservative measures until this is corrected. Often, no other treatment is needed if stretching is successful. If the heel cord is not tight or stretching has not helped, the second step is a soft arch support for the shoe. University of California Biomechanics Laboratory (UCBL) orthotics are necessary in the few cases that do not respond to above measures.

Surgical

Indicated only for the rare symptomatic cases that do not respond to conservative measures. Surgical intervention includes Evans lateral column lengthening, calcaneal osteotomy, subtalar arthrodesis (Grice procedure), triple arthrodesis, or limited midfoot arthrodesis (Hoke-Miller). Of these, the Evans procedure seems to have the best results.

Treatment aims
Asymptomatic flatfeet need no treatment. The goal of treating symptomatic flexible flatfoot is to alleviate the symptoms.

Prognosis
Nonsurgical treatment is successful as a rule. Consideration of operative intervention is rarely needed.

Follow-up and management
Asymptomatic or successfully treated symptomatic flatfoot may be followed on an as-needed basis.

Key references
1. Evans D: Calcaneovalgus deformity. *J Bone Joint Surg [Br]* 1975, 57:270–278.
2. Mosca. Flexible flatfoot and skewfoot. In *The Child's Foot and Ankle.* Edited by Drennan JC. New York: Raven Press; 1992:355–376.
3. Wenger DR, Mauldin E, Speck G, et al.: Corrective shoes and inserts as treatment for flexible flatfoot in infants and children. *J Bone Joint Surg [Am]* 1989, 71:800–810.

Diagnosis

History
Patients present with pain, swelling, and inability to move the finger. They may report a history of an injection or a penetrating injury. Some report subtle trauma to the finger or just an insect bite. The injury can occur acutely without an obvious inciting event.

Physical findings
Kanavel classically described four cardinal signs in flexor tenosynovitis.

Flexed position of the finger.

Symmetric enlargement of the finger.

Presence of excessive tenderness along the entire flexor tendon sheath.

Pain with passive extension of the involved digit.

The last sign is probably the most valuable. It also occurs early in the infectious process and may be the only sign present.

Imaging and laboratory studies
Diagnosis is made by history and physical examination. Plain radiographs are indicated to rule out a foreign body because many of these infections result from injection or penetrating injuries. Laboratory studies include a complete blood count and erythrocyte sedimentation rate for assessment of the degree of infection.

Complications
The most significant complication from an undiagnosed and improperly treated flexor tenosynovitis is destruction of the entire tendon-gliding mechanism and subsequent tendon necrosis and loss of motion. Persistent infection, uncontrolled infection resulting in loss of the digit or even the hand, and stiffness are other complications. The ulnar bursa or the radial bursa can become involved because of the communication between the flexor tendons and these bursae. The flexor pollicis longus sheath is in continuity with the radial bursa, and the flexor digitorum profundus tendon sheath is in continuity with the ulna bursa.

Differential diagnosis
The diagnosis is usually clear, but the degree of involvement is difficult to assess. It is important to differentiate suppurative flexor tenosynovitis, which requires surgical debridement, from early flexor tenosynovitis. In patients with difficulty in motion, pain, and swelling, tendon rupture and fracture must be ruled out.

Etiology or pathophysiology
The most common cause of flexor tenosynovitis is an injection or penetrating injury. Such an injury can result from a variety of objects, such as a needle, a piece of wood, or a paint gun. Hematogenous seeding has also been reported; this often occurs in patients who have diabetes or are immunocompromised.

Epidemiology
Staphylococcus aureus is the most common offending organism. Infections with *Mycobacterium* and *Clostridium* species have recently been reported. The ring, middle, and index fingers are the digits most commonly involved.

Treatment

Nonsurgical

If the diagnosis is made early, usually within 24 to 48 hours of symptom onset, nonsurgical treatment may be attempted. This treatment involves immobilization of the affected hand in a compressive dressing with a splint and then elevation. Empiric intravenous antibiotic therapy should started. A first-generation cephalosporin is sufficient unless the patient is diabetic or immunocompromised. In such patients, additional antibiotics may be indicated. The choice should be determined from the history, clinical findings, and cultures, if obtained. If symptoms do not resolve or improve within 48 hours, surgery should be performed.

Surgical

Surgical debridement is indicated for obvious purulence in the sheath, if the diagnosis is made late, or if early tenosynovitis has not responded to appropriate antibiotics within 48 hours. Many operative techniques have been described. Open drainage may be accomplished through a midaxial incision. Small incisions have also been used to perform irrigation and to instill antibiotics into the sheath via catheters. All patients require antibiotics in addition to surgical irrigation and debridement. Empiric therapy with a first-generation cephalosporin is used. Other antibiotics may be used according to the patient's medical problems and the final results from the intraoperative culture.

Exercise and activity modification

See Nonsurgical treatment section.

Treatment aims
To eradicate the infection, minimize the morbidity associated with the disease process, and prevent loss of motion.

Prognosis
If the diagnosis is made early, nonoperative treatment yields excellent results. If surgery is required, some stiffness remains and the overall prognosis varies from fair to good.

Follow-up and management
All patients require intravenous antibiotics until most of the infection is resolved. Once the symptoms have subsided and the wound (if surgical intervention took place) is free of purulence, intravenous antibiotics may be switched to oral medications. The duration of oral treatment should be 10 to 14 days but can vary depending on the bacteria and the patient's comorbid conditions.

Key references
1. Neviaser RJ: Tenosynovitis. *Hand Clin* 1989, 5:525–53.

Diagnosis

Definition
Fractures about the hip most commonly occur through the femoral neck and intertrochanteric region. Fractures of the acetabulum and the femoral head also occur but are much less common.

History
History of a fall with a blow over the greater trochanter. Most instances involve minor trauma. Stress fractures may have a history of cyclic trauma and an aching about the hip. Major trauma involves a blow along the shaft of the femur.

Physical findings
Affected leg is in external rotation, is abducted, and is slightly shorter than the contralateral limb. Movement elicits crepitus and extreme pain.

Imaging and laboratory studies
Routine radiographs will demonstrate the fracture readily. In cases of minimally displaced fractures in patients with persistent hip pain but no apparent abnormality, magnetic resonance imaging of the affected hip is the best way to detect occult fractures that may later displace.

Complications
Loss of vascularity of femoral head if a minimally displaced fracture is totally displacement.

Osteonecrosis of the femoral head.

Deformity or nonunion if not treated surgically.

20% of young patients with a femoral neck fracture caused by trauma have an ipsilateral femoral shaft fracture.

Differential diagnosis
Dislocation of the hip.
Acetabular fracture.
Stress fracture of the pubic ramus.

Etiology or pathophysiology
Osteoporosis in older age groups.
Trauma in younger populations.
Stress fractures.
When the femoral neck is fractured, the intraosseous cervical vessels are disrupted, leaving the remaining retinacular vessels to provide blood supply to the femoral head.

Classification (Garden)
Garden I—incomplete or impacted fracture of the femoral neck.
Garden II—complete neck fracture without displacement.
Garden III—complete neck fracture with partial displacement.
Garden IV—complete neck fracture with total displacement (Fig. 1).

Epidemiology
250,000 hip fractures per year in the United States alone.

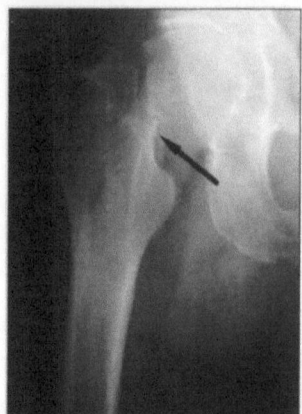

Figure 1. Anteroposterior (AP) radiograph of a hip demonstrating a Garden IV fracture of the right hip (arrow).

Treatment

Nonsurgical
May be indicated for Garden I fractures that are impacted and nondisplaced and have been present for several weeks in an otherwise cooperative patient.
Preoperative treatment consists of longitudinal Buck's traction and bed rest.

Surgical
Pinning with cannulated screws for nondisplaced or minimally displaced fractures and for displaced fractures in younger patients.
Sliding hip screw with side plate for intertrochanteric fractures.
Hemiarthroplasty for displaced fractures in older patients.

Exercise and activity modification
The patient should undergo weight-bearing with crutches as prescribed by the treating physician. Patients usually are able to progress to full weight-bearing within 4 to 6 weeks after fracture, depending on the nature of the fracture and on patient strength. Full weight-bearing usually is tolerated well.

Treatment aims
To preserve the vascularity of the femoral head and restore patient to preinjury ambulatory status.

Prognosis
Nonunion in 15% of cases.
Osteonecrosis in 12% of cases.
Elderly patients generally lose one level of ambulation: if they walked with no aids before the fracture, they will use a cane; if they walked with a cane before, they will use a walker afterward.

Follow-up and management
Evaluation and treatment for osteoporosis in the elderly.
Routine evaluation of fracture healing with radiographs to check for displacement of hardware.

Key references
1. DeLee JC: Fractures and dislocations of the hip. In *Rockwood and Green's Fractures in Adults.* Edited by Rockwood CA, Greene D, Bucholz R. Philadelphia: Lippincott–Raven; 1996:1659–1825.2
2. Kyle RF, Cabanela ME, Russell TA, *et al.*: Fractures of the proximal part of the femur. In *Instructional Course Lectures.* Edited by Jackson DW. Rosemont, IL: American Academy of Orthopaedic Surgeons; 1995:227–254.

Diagnosis

History

Frozen shoulder, also known as adhesive capsulitis, is a diagnosis of exclusion that is characterized clinically by pain and restricted motion. The pain is insidious in onset and is usually noted in the deltoid, with distal radiation to the region of the elbow. Moderate to severe night pain is common. The natural history of frozen shoulder involves three phases: pain, restricted motion, and gradual improvement.

Physical findings

Restricted shoulder motion in all directions.

Strength, stability, and smoothness of joint motion are within normal limits.

Moderate to severe pain is noted when patient attempts to passively move the shoulder beyond the restricted range of active motion.

Imaging and laboratory studies

Routine radiographs (anteroposterior and axillary lateral) are typically normal but should always be obtained to rule out other causes of shoulder stiffness.

Complications

Although frozen shoulder is generally a self-limiting disease, functional limitations and discomfort may persist beyond 5 years.

Fractures of the humerus, glenohumeral dislocation, and brachial plexus palsy have occurred with manipulation under anesthesia (one treatment commonly recommended for persistent frozen shoulder).

Differential diagnosis
Rotator cuff rupture.
Posterior shoulder dislocation.
Cervical disk disease.
Pancoast tumor.

Etiology or pathophysiology
The cause is probably multifactorial, involving inflammatory cells, autoimmune mechanism, and humeral mediators. Tissue contracture may result from interaction among cytokines, inflammatory cell products, and platelet-derived growth factor.

Epidemiology
Incidence of frozen shoulder in the general population is 2%.
Incidence among patients with diabetes mellitus is 10% to 20% (may be up to 40% in insulin-dependent patients).
Higher incidence is also noted with thyroid disorders, cardiac disease, pulmonary conditions, and neoplastic disorders.

Treatment

Nonsurgical

Moist heat, nonsteroidal anti-inflammatory medication, and, occasionally, a mild narcotic to control pain.

Pendulum and gentle, passive stretching exercises using the contralateral arm for motor power (moist heat is applied for 20 minutes before stretching).

Shoulders are moved to the point of feeling a stretching sensation and never to the point of pain (exercises are facilitated with the use of a 3-foot stick and an overhead pulley, with the patient controlling the shoulder range of motion).

Surgical

Manipulation under general anesthesia.

Arthroscopic capsular release.

Open capsular release.

Combined manipulation, open, and arthroscopic capsular release.

Treatment aims

Gradual improvement of shoulder motion and function in the absence of pain. "No pain, no gain" axiom should not be applied.

Prognosis

Prognosis for functional recovery is good, but some stiffness or mild pain may persist.

Recovery may take in excess of 5 years, although many patients improve within 2 years.

Follow-up and management (or rehabilitation).

Stretching program emphasizing flexion and internal and external rotation. Sustained stretching is emphasized (5 to 10 count).

If pain is noted, the patient decreases the intensity of the exercises but maintains a frequency of 3 to 4 times a day.

Key references

1. Miller MD, Wirth MA, Rockwood CA Jr: Thawing the frozen shoulder: the "patient" patient. *Orthopedics* 1996, 19:849–853.

2. Neviaser JS: Adhesive capsulitis and the stiff and painful shoulder. *Orthop Clin North Am* 1980, 11:327–331.

3. Rockwood CA Jr: Management of patients with frozen shoulder. In *Instructional Course Lectures*. Rosemont, IL: American Association of Orthopaedic Surgeons; 1987.

GANGLION OF THE FINGER   A. Agarwal

Diagnosis

History

Patients present with a mass on the volar or dorsal aspect of the finger. Most patients are concerned with the appearance of the mass or with a recent increase in the size of the mass. The mass may be painful, and the onset may be gradual or insidious; trauma does not usually precede its development. Patients may report fluctuations in the size of the mass.

Physical findings

The mass is occasionally tender to palpation. It can either be fixed or mobile and often is firm. Transillumination aids in the diagnosis. The mass is more frequently located on the volar surface of the finger than on the dorsum.

Imaging and laboratory studies

Plain radiographs help exclude associated bony abnormality. Usually, however, the diagnosis is a clinical one and diagnostic studies are not indicated. Magnetic resonance imaging may be useful if the diagnosis is in question.

Complications

The main complication associated with a ganglion of the finger is recurrence.

Differential Diagnosis

Soft tissue tumors about the fingers often mimic a ganglion. In patients with osteoarthritis or rheumatoid arthritis, nodules on the fingers associated with the disease process may resemble ganglions.

Etiology or pathophysiology

The ganglion on a finger originates from the retinacular sheath when it occurs on the volar surface. Dorsal finger ganglions originate from the extensor tendon, usually over the metacarpal.

Epidemiology (see also Ganglion of the Wrist)

Ganglion cysts account for 50% to 70% of soft tissue tumors of the hand and wrist in both children and adults. The female-to-male ratio is 2:1. Of ganglions occurring in the upper extremity, 70% are present on the dorsum of the wrist. Ganglions of the finger account for a small percentage of the overall number of ganglions. Approximately 10% arise from the volar surface of the digit. When they do occur in fingers, the index or ring finger is usually involved. Dorsal finger lesions are rare because ganglions occurring on the dorsum of the hand represent only 2% of all ganglions.

Treatment

Nonsurgical

If the lesion is asymptomatic, reassuring the patient is all that may be needed. Aspiration of the lesion has been shown to be effective. The ganglion is injected with a steroid solution at the time of aspiration to cause scarring of the inner lining; this helps prevent recurrence. Rest, immobilization, and traumatic rupture are ineffective.

Surgical

The surgical option is to excise the lesion, whether on the volar or dorsal surface. This may be indicated for ganglions that affect finger mobility or are painful.

Exercise and activity modification

None.

Treatment Aims

If pain and mobility are of concern, the goal is to provide pain-free mobility of the involved finger. Often, the goal is to reassure the patient that the mass is not cancer.

Prognosis

The overall success rate with surgical treatment is excellent, and recurrence rates are low. Aspiration with steroid injection is 85% successful. Failure of aspiration can be subsequently treated with surgical excision. Therefore, the long-term prognosis for all ganglions of the finger is excellent.

Follow-up and management

After aspiration of a ganglion, immediate motion is allowed. No splinting is required. Immediate postsurgical splinting may be used for 3 to 5 days. After this time, active use of the finger and hand is encouraged.

Key references

1. Richman JA, Gelberman RH, Engber WD, et al.: Ganglions of the wrist and digits: results of treatment by aspiration and cyst wall puncture. J Hand Surg 1987, 12:1041–1043.
2. Diao E, Moy OJ: Common tumors. Orthop Clin North Am 1992, 23:187–196.

Diagnosis

Natural history of physiologic angular deformities

The normal progression of physiologic bowlegs (genu varum) and knock-knees (genu valgum) is age-dependent (Fig. 1). From birth, a child has physiologic bowlegs. This usually corrects by 18 to 24 months of age. A physiologic valgus then occurs, peaking by 36 to 48 months of age. Adult values are achieved by 7 years of age.

History

It is important to note whether the deformity is improving or worsening.

There should be no symptoms on presentation of physiologic angular deformities.

Pain may denote pathologic condition.

Check for family history of the deformity.

Physical findings

Physiologic angular deformities are bilateral and symmetric. Unilateral or asymmetric presentation should be suspicious for pathology. It is important to note whether there is a lateral thrust (genu varum) or medial thrust (genu valgum) because these conditions denote laxity of collateral ligaments. When lax, these ligaments cannot withstand the angular moment about the knee. This is unusual in physiologic conditions and may denote a pathologic condition.

Assess the patient for internal tibial torsion, which may accentuate apparent bowlegs, and pes planus, which will accentuate a knock-knee deformity.

Imaging and laboratory studies

Radiographs: A standing anteroposterior radiograph from the hips to the ankles with knees facing forward is the standard radiograph used to assess angular deformity. Blount's disease presents radiographically with depression of the medial tibial epiphysis and beaking of the medial proximal tibial metaphysis. A metaphyseal diaphyseal angle greater than 11° is highly suggestive of Blount's disease. Other causes of pathologic angular deformity, such as rickets, tumors, or bone dysplasias, should be readily apparent radiologically.

Laboratory studies: Blood chemistries, calcium, phosphate, and vitamin D levels will help differentiate among the various forms of rickets.

Differential diagnosis

Blount's disease: the most common cause of pathologic bowlegs in young children. It can be infantile (occurring in children age 1 to 3.5 years) or adolescent (occurring in children age 8 to 14 years) in onset. Infantile Blount's disease is usually bilateral and progressive. Adolescent Blount's disease is a separate entity. It is unilateral and slowly progressive and presents with knee pain.

Metabolic bone disease (ie, rickets, renal failure): causes either varus or valgus deformity depending on the anatomic alignment at the onset to the condition. Vitamin D–resistant rickets has an early onset and will accentuate physiologic genu varum, whereas renal osteodystrophy develops later in life and usually produces knock-knee deformity.

Infection, tumors (enchondroma) trauma, or bone dysplasias: can affect physeal growth and cause angular deformity.

Proximal tibial metaphyseal fractures: can cause progressive genu valgum through unknown mechanisms. The resultant valgus can be significant (up to 25°) but usually spontaneously resolves with growth. Early osteotomies tend to again stimulate asymmetric growth and lead to recurrence of the valgus deformity.

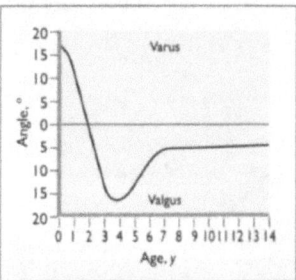

Treatment

Nonsurgical

Most cases of angular deformity are physiologic and spontaneously resolve. The parents of the patient will need reassurance and support. Ambulatory brace treatment is effective in correcting early infantile Blount's disease. Treatment may last from 1 to 2 years.

Surgical

Late infantile or adolescent Blount's disease must be treated by corrective angular osteotomy. The internal tibial torsion associated with infantile form of the disease should also be corrected. For the most advanced cases, physeal bar resection or elevation of the medial tibial plateau may be needed. Severe genu valgum persisting into adolescence or the teen years can be treated with medial proximal tibial or distal femoral stapling, hemiepiphysiodesis, or osteotomy.

Surgical complications after proximal tibial osteotomy include compartment syndrome of the leg and recurrence of varus deformity. Fasciotomy of the anterior and lateral compartments is recommended at the time of osteotomy, and careful postoperative observation is warranted to avoid a compartment syndrome.

Treatment aims
To correct pathologic angular deformities.

Prognosis
The prognosis depends on the cause and severity of the deformity.

Follow-up and management
If no abnormality is noted, it is usually helpful to suggest that the parents obtain standing photographs of the child from the front and from behind. These pictures are compared with the child's appearance 4 to 6 months later. If no improvement is noticeable, the parents should call for a follow-up appointment. Infantile Blount's disease that is successfully treated with a brace should not recur; only one or two follow-up examinations in the year after bracing are necessary. Surgically corrected angular deformities should be followed closely for several years to monitor for recurrence.

Key references

1. Bowen JR, Leahey JL, Zhang ZH: Partial epi-physiodesis at the knee to correct angular deformity. *Clin Orthop* 1985, 198:194–190.
2. Kling TF: Angular deformities of the lower limbs in children. *Orthop Clin North Am* 1987, 18:513–127.
3. Tolo VT: The lower extremity. In *Lovell and Winters's Pediatric Orthopedics.* Edited by Morrissy RT, Weinstein SL. Philadelphia: Lippincott–Raven: 1996:1054–1061.
4. Zionts LE, MacEwen GD: Spontaneous improvement of post-traumatic tibia valga. *J Bone Joint Surg* 1986, 68A:680–686.

Diagnosis

Definition
Known as "the disease of kings and the king of diseases," gout is the result of tissue deposition of crystals of monosodium urate from supersaturated extracellular fluids.

History
Acute arthritis is the most common early clinical manifestation; 75% of cases involve the metatarsophalangeal joint of the great toe. Early attacks subside over 3 to 10 days, even without treatment. The first episode usually occurs abruptly in a single joint in the middle of the night so that the patient awakens with dramatic unexplained joint pain and swelling.

Physical findings
The first metatarsophalangeal joint is most commonly involved, but the ankle, tarsal area, and the knee are also commonly involved.

Imaging and laboratory studies
Joint aspirate demonstrates needle-like crystals that are negatively birefringent when using a polarizing microscope.

Synovial fluid leukocyte count between 20,000 and 100,000 cells/mm^3.

Serum urate level is of limited value and may be normal even during gouty attack.

24-h urine uric acid can be used for assessing the risk for renal stones. Urinary excretion greater than 750 to 1000 mg of uric acid per day suggests overproduction.

Complications
Recurrent attacks of severe arthritis.

Accumulation of crystalline deposits (tophi).

Renal impairment (gouty nephropathy).

Uric acid calculi in the urinary tract.

Osteonecrosis of the hip.

Differential diagnosis
Infection.
Pseudogout.
Fracture.

Etiology or pathophysiology
Gout is caused by an excess of uric acid in the body. This excess can be caused by an increase in production by the body, by underelimination of uric acid by the kidneys, or by increased intake of foods containing purines, which are metabolized to uric acid in the body. Certain meats, seafood, dried peas, and beans are particularly high in purines. Alcoholic beverages may also significantly increase uric acid levels and precipitate gout attacks.

Epidemiology
Predominantly affects men.
Peak incidence in fifth decade of life.
Incidence in men: 13.6/1000; incidence in women: 6.4/1000.

Treatment

Nonsurgical

Short-term: Nonsteroidal anti-inflammatory drugs: Indomethacin, 150 mg, for the first dose, followed by 50 mg every 8 hours. Monitor for gastrointestinal involvement. May use colchicine, 0.05 mg, 1 or 2 tablets initially followed by 1 tablet every hour until symptoms subside or gastrointestinal side effects occur. Neither of these medications affects urate levels.

Aspirate the joint for diagnosis and relief of symptoms from swelling.

Splint the affected joint.

Use analgesics for pain control.

Long-term: Allopurinol (xanthine oxidase inhibitor): 100 to 300 mg/d or probenecid (increases urate excretion).

One or other of the anti-inflammatory drugs can be effective; however, to gain the best results, the dose should be adequate and the drug taken as soon as possible at the first sign of an attack. Thus, medical advice must be sought early. With effective treatment, the attack may be controlled within 12 to 24 hours and treatment need not be continued after a few days. Rest and elevation of the part involved and fluid intake increased by an extra 4 or 5 glasses of water a day are also important. Drugs used for the acute attack have no effect on reducing uric acid levels.

Surgical

There is no surgical treatment for gout but surgery may be indicated in the treatment of avascular necrosis of the hip.

Exercise and activity modification

Behavioral modification of the diet is necessary. Patients must reduce or eliminate foods that are high in purines. See Treatment aims section.

Treatment aims

Whenever possible, the first step must be to correct the factors that give rise to high uric acid levels. The following foods, which are high in purines, should be restricted or avoided:
Liver, kidneys, tripe, sweetbreads, and tongue.
Red meat.
Shellfish, fish roe, and scallops.
Peas, lentils, and beans.
Alcohol, especially beer and wine.

Prognosis

Best results are obtained when treatment begins early in the course of the disease. Diet control can significantly reduce symptoms. Chronic attacks can damage cartilage and lead to arthritis.

Follow-up and management

Indomethacin for up to 1 week for acute attacks. Allopurinol for long-term management. Increased fluid intake is important.

Key references

1. *Primer on the Rheumatic Diseases* edn 10. Edited by Schumacher HR. Atlanta: The Arthritis Foundation; 1993.

Diagnosis

Definition
Also known as "greater trochanteric pain syndrome," greater trochanteric bursitis is characterized by tenderness and pain over the region of the greater trochanter of the hip.

History
Pain radiates down the lateral aspect of the leg as far as the ankle but not into the foot. Patients cannot sleep on the affected side and report that the pain is worse when they arise from bed or a seated position. Pain improves after several steps but returns after ambulation lasting more than 30 minutes.

Trochanteric bursitis may occur with other problems, including leg length inequality, previous surgical fixation of the hip, spinal disorders, and rheumatoid arthritis. Most patients report symptoms lasting from several months to years.

Physical findings
Point tenderness over the greater trochanter in more than 90% of all patients presenting with trochanteric bursitis.

Trendelenburg's sign (dropping of the pelvis to the contralateral side when standing on the affected hip).

Normal range of motion unless associated with other hip abnormality. Painless internal rotation. May have pain with flexion and external rotation. Pain can be reproduced with extension, adduction, and external rotation, which rubs the trochanter against the iliotibial band.

Imaging and laboratory studies
Radiography (anteroposterior and lateral) of hip to rule out other abnormalities. Radiographs should appear normal, although irregularities about the trochanter may be apparent in 27% to 40% of cases.

Diagnostic injection of the greater trochanteric bursa with lidocaine and corticosteroid. Immediate relief suggests local bursitis.

Complications
Limp.

Chronic pain.

Differential diagnosis
Osteoarthritis of the hip: usually associated with painful internal rotation.
Sciatica: neurologic changes may occur.
Trochanteric fracture: especially in cases of osteoporosis or associated with total hip arthroplasty.

Etiology
Inflammation of overlying bursa of greater trochanter, possibly from overuse or blunt trauma.

Epidemiology
May occur in any age group but is predominant in middle-aged and older groups.

Treatment

Nonsurgical

Nonsteroidal anti-inflammatory drugs.

Stretching exercises of the iliotibial band.

Local infiltration of the bursa with lidocaine and steroid.

Surgical

Surgical intervention is rarely indicated and should be considered only after a thorough diagnostic evaluation has ruled out other potential sources of pain in the area. Removal of prominent metallic hardware may relieve symptoms.

Exercise and activity modification

The patient should use stretching exercises for the iliotibial band.

Treatment aims
To reduce inflammation and relieve tension on the iliotibial band.

Prognosis
All patients responded to one (71%), two (22%), or three injections (7%). Symptoms recurred in only 8% after 17 months [1].

Follow-up and management
Follow-up as symptoms dictate with nonsteroidal anti-inflammatory drugs, injections, and exercise.

Key references
1. Berry DJ: Soft tissue disorders. In *The Adult Hip.* Edited by Callaghan JJ, Rosenberg AG, Rubash HE. Philadelphia: Lippincott–Raven; 1998:593–600.
2. Snider RK: *Essentials of Musculoskeletal Care.* Rosemont, IL: American Academy of Orthopaedic Surgeons; 1997.

Diagnosis

History

Patient reports pain over the dorsum of the proximal interphalangeal joint of the affected toe, where the deformed digit has been rubbing on the shoe. A hard corn develops over the dorsum of the proximal interphalangeal joint in response to long-term shoe irritation. This area of hyperkeratotic skin becomes so thick that it makes the hammertoe even more easily irritated by tight shoewear. A painful callus may develop under the tip of the toe or under the respective metatarsal head.

Physical findings

Hammertoe is characterized by hyperextension of the metatarsophalangeal joint, a flexion contracture of the proximal interphalangeal joint, and hyperextension of the distal interphalangeal joint. The deformity is accentuated by weight-bearing active extension of the toes (Fig. 1). Often, a tender corn can be identified on the dorsum of the proximal interphalangeal joint.

Imaging and laboratory studies

Standing anteroposterior and lateral radiographs of the forefoot show the bony deformity. The metatarsophalangeal joint may rarely be dislocated and the proximal phalanx will be riding on the dorsal neck of the metatarsal.

Complications

In patients with peripheral neuropathy, such as that occurring in diabetes, the pressure on the dorsum of the proximal interphalangeal joint can cause ulceration and infection.

Differential diagnosis

Hammertoes should be distinguished from clawtoes. A clawtoe deformity is very similar but also features a flexion deformity of the distal interphalangeal joint. With clawtoes, the hyperextension deformity of the metatarsophalangeal joint is usually much more severe and is usually fixed.

Etiology or pathophysiology

Hammertoes have many causes. Subtle muscle imbalances between the intrinsic and extrinsic musculature of the foot can lead to this deformity. Tight shoewear aggravates the problem. As the deformity progresses, the extrinsic tendons become contracted and the deformities become fixed.

Epidemiology

Hammertoes usually occur in adults. They are seen more commonly in women than in men, in part because of a hereditary predisposition and wearing of high-heeled, pointed-toed shoes.

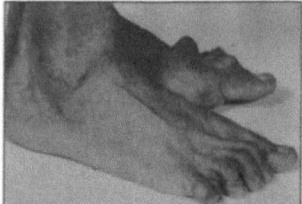

Figure 1. Hammertoe deformities of the right second, third, and fourth toes.

Treatment

Nonsurgical

Treatment of symptoms is directed at relieving the shoe pressure over the painful corn on the dorsum of the proximal interphalangeal joint. This goal can be accomplished by wearing shoes with an extra-depth toe box and providing padding for the bony prominences. Thickened corns and calluses should be regularly trimmed or sanded to keep them from getting too large.

Surgical

Surgical treatment should be limited to patients who do not respond to nonoperative management. A variety of different surgical approaches have been described, all of which focus on correcting the deformities and rebalancing the soft tissues to prevent recurrence. These goals often necessitate resection of bone (usually the head of the proximal phalanx) and release of the soft tissues, particularly the extensor tendons and the dorsal capsule of the metatarsophalangeal joint. Some authors recommend fusion of the proximal interphalangeal joint to secure a long-term correction, particularly in young persons. Other authors have recommended flexor to extensor tendon transfers to rebalance the dynamic forces acting on the digit.

Treatment aims
To relieve pain and prevent the development of ulcerations over the dorsum of the proximal interphalangeal joint .

Prognosis
Hammertoe is usually amenable to treatment. The symptoms should be controlled so that the patient can participate in as vigorous an active lifestyle.

Follow-up and management
Hammertoe deformities can recur, particularly if patients resume wearing high-heeled, pointed-toed shoes. Everyone should be encouraged to wear sensible shoewear at all times.

Key references

1. Meyerson MS, Shereff MJ: The pathologic anatomy of claw and hammertoes. *J Bone Joint Surg* 1989, 71:45–49.
2. Mizel MS, Yodlwski ML: Disorders of the lesser metatarsophalangeal joints. *J Am Acad Orthop Surg* 1995, 3:166–173.

Diagnosis

History
Humeral shaft fracture usually results from a direct impact to the arm. It can also be caused by an indirect injury in which the deforming force is applied through the forearm or hand.

Physical findings
Deformity of the arm, swelling, ecchymosis, or bruising.

Crepitance or motion at the fracture site with palpation.

Possibly diminished distal pulses or nerve deficits.

Imaging and laboratory studies
Plain radiographs of the shoulder and elbow joints should be obtained (Fig. 1). If distal circulation is interrupted, arteriography may be required to discover the location of the vascular disruption.

Complications
Malunion, nonunion, Volkmann's ischemic contracture of the forearm and hand, permanent nerve palsy or paresis (most commonly of the radial nerve).

Differential diagnosis
Arm contusion; shoulder fracture, dislocation, or fracture-dislocation; elbow fracture, dislocation, or fracture-dislocation; vascular injury to the brachial artery or vein; injury to the radial, ulnar, or median nerve.

Etiology or pathophysiology
Falls onto the arm, direct impact from an object, crush injury, arm wrestling.

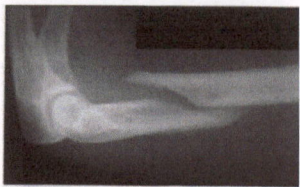

Figure 1. Radiograph of a humeral shaft fracture.

Treatment

Nonsurgical

Most cases are treated with a hanging-arm cast, co-adaptation splint, or functional brace. Early active shoulder and elbow motions are encouraged. Healing generally occurs within 3 months of injury.

Surgical

Surgery is generally the exception rather than the rule. Strong advocates for both intramedullary and plate-and-screws fixation when surgical fixation is employed. With concomitant nerve or vessel injury, the humerus is generally stabilized at the time of surgical repair of the nerve or vessel.

Exercise and activity modification

Smoking is a significant factor in the failure of humeral fractures to heal normally.

Treatment aims

To achieve a solidly united humerus with little angulatory, rotational, or axial malalignment.

To achieve full active motion in the elbow and shoulder.

To achieve normal vascular and neural function in the forearm and hand distal to the injury.

Prognosis

Within 6 months of injury, the prognosis for complete return of function in a closed fracture is good. If the fracture is associated with a vascular or nerve injury, recovery of function is usually delayed and incomplete. Open fractures may even necessitate amputation.

Follow-up and management

For closed fractures treated nonoperatively, intermittent follow-up should be done for at least 6 months to monitor healing and return of function. Fractures treated operatively should be followed in a similar manner but should also be assessed for operative complications, such as infection and implant failure. Nerve injuries occurring in closed fractures should generally be observed for return of function. Open injuries resulting in nerve dysfunction should be explored at the time of fracture debridement for evidence of nerve injury or transection.

Key references

1. Holm CL: Management of humeral shaft fractures. *Clin Orthop Rel Res* 1970, 71:132–139. 2

2. Packer JW, Foster RR, Garcia A, Grantham SA: The humeral fracture with radial nerve palsy: is exploration warranted? *Clin Orthop* 1972, 34–38.

3. Sarmiento A, Kinman PB, Galvin EG, et al.: Functional bracing of fractures of the shaft of the humerus. *J Bone Joint Surg [Am]* 1977, 59:596–601.

P. Jacobs

Diagnosis

History
Chronic repetitive irritation.
Insidious onset.
Pain, especially with overhead activities.
Weakness.
Night pain/difficulty sleeping on shoulder.
Pain with forward flexion and internal rotation.

Physical findings
Tenderness localized to proximal lateral aspect of the humerus.
Normal to slightly decreased range of motion, although with pain.
Increased pain with arc of forward elevation from 70° to 120°.
Atrophy of shoulder girdle in chronic cases.
Crepitus: subacromial region (hypertrophy/scarring of subacromial bursa).
Impingement sign: described by Neer; pain occurring on elevation of arm in the forward plane with humerus internally rotated and stabilizing the scapula (compress the rotator cuff on undersurface of acromion).
Hawkins sign: pain with 90° of forward flexion with forced internal rotation (drives greater tuberosity under coracoacromial ligament).
Important to document rotator cuff strength (supraspinatus, subscapularis, infraspinatus/teres minor).

Laboratory and imaging studies
Plain radiographs:
Anteroposterior: glenohumeral joint.
Outlet view: structure of acromion.
Axillary lateral: anterior acromial projection; os acromiale.
30° caudal tilt: subacromial spur/excrescence.
Magnetic resonance imaging: not useful except to rule out rotator cuff tear.

Complications
Associated with operative treatment:
Acromial fracture.
Infection.
Inadequate decompression/bone resection (recurrence).
Neurovascular injury.
Deltoid detachment.
Rotator cuff tear.

Differential diagnosis
Biceps tendinitis.
Glenohumeral instability.
Cervical radiculopathy.
Brachial plexopathy.
Acromioclavicular arthritis.
Os acromiale.
Glenohumeral osteoarthritis.
Rotator cuff tear.
Proximal humerus/shoulder girdle tumor.
Pancoast tumor.
Cholecystitis.

Etiology or pathophysiology
Structural factors.
Acromial shape.
Type I: flat (17% of cases).
Type II: curved (43% of cases).
Type III: hooked (40% of cases).
Osteophytes of acromioclavicular joint.
Hypertrophy and enthesopathy of coracoacromial ligament.
Os acromiale.
Malunion of fractures (greater tuberosity, distal clavicle or acromion).
Inflammatory bursitis.
Calcific tendinitis.
Bursal side partial-thickness rotator cuff tear.
Dynamic factors: injury to rotator cuff.
Repetitive microtrauma.
Weakness in rotator cuff allows superior humeral head migration with impingement.
Neer described 3 stages of impingement:
Stage 1: edema/hemorrhage.
Stage 2: tendinitis and fibrosis.
Stage 3: tendon degeneration/rotator cuff tear.

Epidemiology
Increased incidence with occupations or sports associated with repetitive overhead activities.
In one study, 70% of rotator cuff tears had Type III acromion.

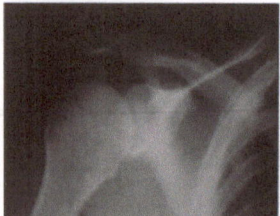
Figure 1. Radiograph of 30° caudal tilt shows subacromial spur.

Treatment

Nonsurgical

Physical therapy/rehabilitation program for 3 months (range of motion/stretching/strengthening).

Prevent overuse/reinjury.

Maintain range of motion/minimize immobility (avoid frozen shoulder).

Nonsteroidal anti-inflammatory drugs.

Hot and cold therapy.

Ultrasonography.

Subacromial injection used for both diagnosis and therapy; lidocaine, marcaine, celestone; when pain or impingement signs are decreased or eliminated, confirms diagnosis.

Surgical

Indicated if conservative treatment has failed after 3 to 6 months.

Open versus arthroscopic decompression.

With arthroscopic decompression, important to perform arthroscopy of the glenohumeral joint to rule out intra-articular abnormality.

Activity and exercise modification

Eliminate activity that exacerbates symptoms.

Treatment aims

Decrease pain.

Increase range of motion.

Surgical: decompress subacromial space.

Prognosis

80% to 90% of patients with impingement symptoms will respond to conservative therapy.

If surgery is indicated, results are good to excellent in 80% of cases.

Follow-up and management

Important to closely follow patient with significant decrease in range of motion until motion is regained.

More than 3 to 4 subacromial injections a year are not recommended.

Key references

1. Altchek DW, Carson EM: Arthroscopic acromioplasty: indications and technique. In *Instructional Course Lectures* vol 47. Rosemont, IL: American Academy of Orthopaedic Surgeons; 1998:21–28.

2. Bigliani LU, Morrison DS, April EW: The morphology of the acromion and its relationship to rotator cuff tears. *Orthop Trans* 1986, 10:228.

3. Gartsman GM: Arthroscopic acromioplasty for lesions of the rotator cuff. *J Bone Joint Surg [Am]* 1990, 72:169–180.

4. Hawkins RJ, Kennedy JC: Impingement syndrome in athletes. *Am J Sports Med* 1980, 8:151–158.

5. Morrison DS, Bigliani LU: Roentgenographic analysis of acromial morphology and its relationship to rotator cuff tears. *Orthop Trans* 1987, 11:439.

6. Neer CS II: Anterior acromioplasty for chronic impingement syndrome in the shoulder: a preliminary report. *J Bone Joint Surg [Am]* 1972, 54:41–50.

7. Seltzer OG, Wirth MA, Rockwood CA: Complications and failures of open and arthroscopic acromioplasties. *Operative Techniques in Sports Medicine* 1994, 2:136–150.

Diagnosis

History

Ingrown toenail usually affects the great toe (Fig. 1), but any digit can be involved. The patient reports pain, redness, swelling, and sometimes purulent drainage from around the periphery of the toenail. The pain is aggravated by shoewear or pressure from any source.

Physical findings

The nail fold is swollen, red, and exquisitely tender to palpation. Hypertrophic granulation tissue is found overlying the nail, and seropurulent drainage often occurs from beneath the granulation tissue.

Imaging and laboratory studies

Radiographs of the digit usually are normal. A chronic infection may rarely have spread to the underlying bone. A rare cause of the hypertrophic granulation tissue is not a simple ingrown nail but rather a subungual exostosis that can be seen as a bony spur growing at a right angle away from the distal phalanx directly underneath the nail.

Complications

A chronic ingrown toenail can lead to a persistent infection of the digit and, on rare occasions, can cause osteomyelitis of the underlying distal phalanx. Chronic inflammation and infection can lead to elevation of the nail, producing irregularity and fissuring of the nail itself.

Differential diagnosis

The rare subungual exostosis is sometimes confused with the very common ingrown toenail.

Etiology or pathophysiology

Instead of growing over the nail fold, the lateral or medial edge of the toenail grows into it and causes skin irritation and inflammation. Eventually, a low-grade infection develops. Cutting the toenail in a curved fashion encourages the development of an ingrown toenail. Tight shoewear causes the nail fold to press onto and over the top of the nail, further aggravating the problem.

Epidemiology

Ingrown toenail is common in adolescents but may occur in anyone who cuts the toenails improperly or wears shoes that are too tight.

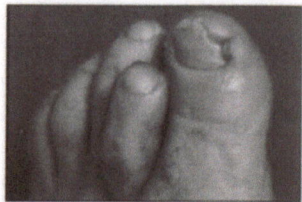

Figure 1. Ingrown toenail on the medial edge of the great toe.

Treatment

Nonsurgical

The early ingrown toenail can be treated effectively by avoiding tight shoewear. An orangewood stick can be used to push the nail fold out over the top of the ingrowing nail edge. A small cotton pledget can be placed under the corner of the nail to hold it up and over the nail fold. The pledget should be changed daily and left in place until the corner of the nail has a chance to grow out over the top of the nail fold.

Surgical

Chronic, recalcitrant ingrown toenail can be treated surgically by partial excision of the toenail, with removal of up to one-third of the width of the nail and all of the lateral and medial edge that has grown up and underneath the nail fold. Most authors recommend that the germinal matrix of this portion of the nail be ablated, either by surgical excision or the application of phenol to the germinal matrix. Doing so prevents recurrent growth of this portion of the nail and creates a narrower toenail that is less likely to grow under the nail fold in the future.

Exercise and activity modification

Proper shoewear should always be worn to minimize the chance of creating an ingrown toenail. An ingrown toenail can often be prevented by proper clipping of the nails. The toenails should be cut transversely rather than in a curved fashion. The transverse cut allows for the edges of the nails to extend out over the nail fold and minimizes the chance of developing an ingrown toenail.

Treatment aims
The goal of treatment is to preserve as much of the great toenail as possible and achieve a stable state where the corner of the nail extends beyond the nail fold.

Prognosis
Generally, the prognosis for an ingrown toenail is excellent.

Follow-up and management
Proper shoewear should always be worn to minimize the chance of recurrence of this problem.

Key references
1. Grieg JD, Anderson JH, Ireland AJ, et al.: The surgical treatment of ingrown toenail. J Bone Joint Surg 1991, 73:131–133.
2. Zuber TJ, Pfenninger JL: Management of ingrown toenails. Am Fam Physician 1995, 52:181–190.

Diagnosis

History
No symptoms are reported with excessive intoeing. The condition is usually first noticed after walking begins. Parents may report that their children trip or fall more often than usual.

Physical findings
A rotational profile should be made for each body segment. Measure the foot-progression angle, hip rotation, and tibial rotation (thigh-foot angle or the transmalleolar axis) and note any foot deformity such as metatarsus adductus. Assess the gait pattern. Medial femoral torsion is seen when the patella are medially rotated with the feet during gain. The patella are straightforward, and only the feet are inturned with internal tibial torsion. Also assess neurologic status.

Imaging and laboratory studies
Radiographs: Rarely needed unless hip dysplasia or other problems are suspected.

Complications
There are no proven long-term effects from excessive intoeing into adult life.

Differential diagnosis
Internal tibial torsion.
Medial femoral torsion.
Metatarsus adductus.
Cerebral palsy or other neuromuscular disease, which may present with abnormal lower-extremity rotation.

Etiology or pathophysiology
Metatarsus adductus and internal tibial torsion are a product of intrauterine positioning.
Sleeping or sitting positions may delay or prevent resolution of the deformity. Sitting with the feet turned in under the buttocks delays resolution of internal tibial torsion. Sitting in the "W" position delays improvement of femoral anteversion or medial femoral torsion.
Rotation is considered abnormal if it differs by more than 2 standard deviations from the mean.

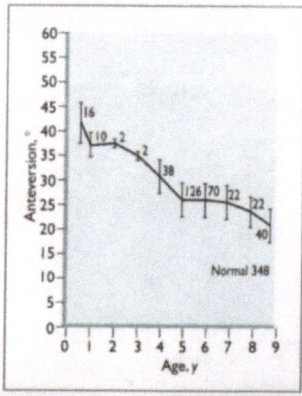

Figure 1. Femoral anteversion spontaneously improves through early childhood. (*From* Crane L: Femoral torsion and its relation to toeing-in and toeing-out. *J Bone Joint Surg [Am]* 1959, 41:423.)

Treatment

Nonsurgical

Nighttime bracing for internal tibial torsion is effective. Because most cases spontaneously improve, the Denis-Browne bar should be reserved for patients followed for 9 to 12 months without any improvement. No bracing or orthotic is effective for improving excessive medial femoral torsion.

Surgical

Operative intervention for internal tibial or medial femoral torsion should not be undertaken before age 7 years because until that time, improvement is highly likely. A supramalleolar osteotomy is preferable for internal tibial torsion. Femoral derotation osteotomy can be accomplished in the subtrochanteric or supracondylar level. Surgical complications include compartment syndrome and inadvertent angular deformities.

Treatment aims
To correct pathologic internal rotation to normal values.

Prognosis
Most rotational deformities in infants and young children spontaneously correct by age 3 to 4 years. Adult values are reached by 7 years. Internal tibial torsion is the most common cause for intoeing, and it usually spontaneously improves through age 7 years. Femoral anteversion gradually decreases from 40° at birth to 10° to 15° by age 8 years (Fig. 1).

Follow-up and management
Once a rotational deformity has been corrected by bracing or surgery, follow-up with patients as needed.

Key References
1. Staheli LT: Rotational problems of the lower extremities. *Orthop Clin North Am* 1987, 18:503–512.
2. Tolo VT: The lower extremity. In *Lovell and Winter's Pediatric Orthopedics.* Edited by Morrissy RT, Weinstein SL. Philadelphia: Lippincott–Raven; 1996:1047–1054.

J.D. Heckman

Diagnosis

History

Sprain of the lateral ankle ligament complex, one of the most common musculo-skeletal injuries, can result from a twisting injury in an athletic event or simply by missing a step. Patients usually report an acute episode of giving way of the ankle with the foot turning inward. Following the initial event are acute pain, swelling, and ecchymosis, usually along the lateral border of the ankle and foot (Fig. 1). Weight bearing is often difficult if not impossible. The patients can sometimes take a few steps, but the pain and swelling then become more severe, further limiting weight bearing.

Physical findings

The acutely sprained ankle is swollen, and active range of motion is limited because of pain. Often, the area of ligament injury is bruised. The most critical step in the physical examination is to identify point tenderness. Careful palpation with one finger over the prominent bony landmarks identifies injury to the anterior talofibular and the calcaneofibular ligaments. With severe sprains, results on the anterior drawer test (anterior talofibular ligament) and the inversion stress test (calcaneofibular ligament) will be positive, indicating acute, complete injury of the respective stabilizing ligaments. When one suspects a tear of the anterior tibiofibular ligament (the syndesmosis), a "squeeze test" should be performed. Firmly compressing the tibia and fibula together at the level of the mid-leg will cause significant pain over the area of the syndesmosis distally if that is the site of injury.

Imaging and laboratory studies

Anteroposterior, lateral, and mortise radiographs of the ankle should be obtained for most acute ankle injuries. If there is no bony tenderness over the distal 6 cm of the lateral malleolus or the medial malleolus and no tenderness over the navicular or the base of the fifth metatarsal, and the patient can bear full weight on the injured ankle, a bony injury is extremely unlikely. Some authors recommend simple treatment of symptoms while avoiding the expense of radiographs in minimally symptomatic patients with an acute ankle injury. In all other circumstances, radiographs should be obtained. Sprain injuries sometimes cause avulsion of small bony fragments from the tip of the medial or lateral malleolus at the point of origin of the stabilizing ligaments. When complete disruption of the lateral ankle ligament complex is suspected, inversion stress radiographs may demonstrate excessive tilting of the talus in the ankle mortise.

Complications

Complications from an ankle sprain are few. Almost all sprains heal without residual problems. The lateral ligament complex sometimes heals in a lengthened state, leading to chronic laxity and recurrent inversion instability that may need to be treated surgically.

Differential diagnosis

The most commonly injured structures on the lateral side of the ankle are the anterior talofibular and the calcaneofibular ligaments. On occasion, other structures may be injured. It is important to distinguish injury of these two ligaments from a tear of the syndesmosis (the anterior tibiofibular ligament), which can be diagnosed by finding direct tenderness over the ligament and by noting positive results on a squeeze test. Other structures in the same area that can be injured and confused with a lateral ligament sprain are avulsion fracture of the base of the fifth metatarsal, dislocation of the peroneal tendons, avulsion fracture of the lateral process of the talus, and avulsion fracture of the anterior process of the calcaneus. These fractures can all be identified by careful inspection of the ankle radiographs.

Etiology or pathophysiology

Lateral ankle sprain results from forced inversion of the foot, which drives the talus into a varus posture and thus puts tension on the anterior talofibular and fibulocalcaneal ligaments. Usually the anterior talofibular ligament fails first, followed by the fibulocalcaneal ligament. Many individuals have degrees of ligamentous laxity that make them susceptible to recurrent inversion ankle sprains.

Epidemiology

A lateral ligament ankle sprain is one of the most common injuries of the musculoskeletal system.

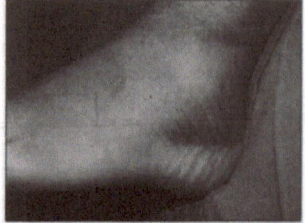

Figure 1. Signs of acute ankle sprain. Note ecchymosis and swelling of the lateral ankle.

Treatment

Nonsurgical

Nonsurgical treatment is based on the severity of the injury. Mild and moderate sprains should be treated with rest, ice, compression, and elevation of the injured limb (RICE). Rest can be accomplished by placing the injured ankle in a supportive splint or boot and giving the patient crutches to use. Ice should be applied for 24 to 48 hours after the acute injury. The ankle can be compressed with an elastic bandage or a supportive splint or boot. To minimize swelling, the foot should be elevated to above the level of the heart for the first 24 hours. Mild sprains respond to this treatment in a few days, allowing a fairly quick return to function. Moderate sprains may require 2 to 3 weeks to recover fully. A severe sprain, one in which both the anterior talofibular and the calcaneofibular ligaments have been torn, may require as long as 6 weeks to heal. Cast immobilization for 2 to 3 weeks immediately after the injury supports the healing tissues once the acute swelling has subsided. An aggressive rehabilitation program should be pursued to restore ankle joint function after all ankle ligament injuries.

Surgical

There is no indication for surgical treatment of an acute lateral ankle ligament sprain.

Treatment aims

To allow the injured ligaments to heal and to restore function as soon as possible.

Prognosis

The prognosis for most lateral ankle sprains is excellent. Most heal without any residual problems. Only a small percentage of injuries heal with residual symptomatic laxity that requires surgical reconstruction.

Rehabilitation

As the acute symptoms subside, patients should engage in aggressive rehabilitation to restore strength and range of motion to the ankle. The most important component of the rehabilitation program should be a focus on strengthening the peroneal muscles and restoring proprioceptive function to the ankle and foot. This can be accomplished best by the use of a BAPS board (Biomechanical Ankle Platform System, Camp International, Jackson, MI).

Key references

1. Holmer P, Sondergaard L, Konradsen L, et al.: Epidemiology of sprains in the lateral ankle and foot. *Foot Ankle* 1994, 15:72–74.
2. Marder RA: Current methods for the evaluation of ankle ligament injuries. *J Bone Joint Surg* 1994, 76:1103–1111.
3. Colville MR: Reconstruction of the lateral ankle ligaments. *J Bone Joint Surg* 1994, 76:1092–1102.

Diagnosis

History

Legg-Calvé-Perthes (LCP) disease is an idiopathic avascular necrosis of the femoral head in children. Patients have a limp that is often associated with hip pain; antecedent trauma and signs of systemic infection are rare. Activity increases hip pain, stiffness, and muscle spasm; rest reduces these symptoms.

Physical findings

In the acute stage, the hip is painful when moved and is tender to palpation. Range of motion is limited by muscle spasm, especially with internal rotation of the hip. The patient holds the hip in flexion and external rotation and guards against hip motion. The limp may be antalgic. The Trendelenberg sign, a lurching to the affected side when the patient performs weight-bearing during gait, is seen on the affected side. a lurching to the affected side when the patient performs weight-bearing during gait. In the fragmentation stage, the hip may have an adduction contracture and could be stiff to both abduction and internal rotation with mild discomfort during passive range of motion.

Imaging and laboratory studies

Anteroposterior radiographs of the pelvis, including the hips, and frog-leg lateral radiographs of both hips should be obtained. In the initial stage of LCP disease, radiographs may be negative or may only show mild widening of the joint space of the hip, increased density of the ossific nucleus of the hip, irregularity of the physis, and radiolucency of the metaphysis. Technetium bone scanning, if the diagnosis is uncertain, may show decreased isotope pick-up of the femoral head. In the fragmentation stage of LCP disease, the epiphysis has areas of dense sclerotic bone and areas of radiolucency. A subchordal fracture over the necrotic area of head is known as the *crescent sign*.

Complications

Coxa magna may develop, in which the lateral portion enlarges to form a saddle-shaped femoral head that can lead to hinged abduction. Premature physeal arrest can centrally shorten the femoral neck. Lateral arrest produces an oval femoral head that is tilted into valgus with greater trochanteric overgrowth; this may require distal trochanteric transfer. Partial physis arrest may cause an irregular femoral head, which may also develop hinge abduction. In 3% of hips, osteochondritis dissecans can occur. Symptomatic hips are treated with fragment drilling, pinning, or excision.

Differential diagnosis

Transient synovitis of the hip.
Bacterial septic arthritis of the hip.
Hemophilia.
Juvenile rheumatoid arthritis.
Lymphoma.
Rheumatic fever.
Traumatic avascular hip necrosis.
Osteomyelitis of the proximal femur.
Osteomyelitis of the pelvis.
Eosinophilic granuloma, lymphoma, osteoblastoma, osteoid osteoma, and chondroblastoma of the proximal femur.
Sickle cell disease.
Gaucher disease.
Hypothyroidism
Bilateral hip involvement: multiple epiphyseal dysplasia or spondylo-epiphyseal dysplasia.

Etiology

The cause of LCP disease is avascular necrosis of the femoral head, but the cause of the vascular compromise is unknown. The most current theory suggests that abnormal blood clotting factors may be involved in the cause of LCP disease, but this theory remains controversial.

Epidemiology

Incidence of LCP disease is 1/1200 in the United States; incidence in Asian, central European, and Eskimo persons is increased. Average age at onset is 6 years (range, 2 to 13 years). The peak age range, involving 80% of patients, is between 4 and 9 years. The ratio of girls to boys is 1:4. Onset age is earlier for girls than for boys. Children with LCP disease have skeletal maturity delayed an average of 21 months and are shorter than average. There are no proven family inheritance factors. The disease is bilateral in about 10% of cases.

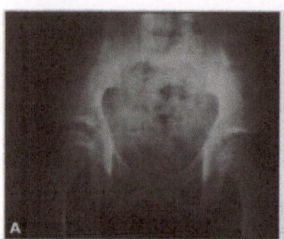
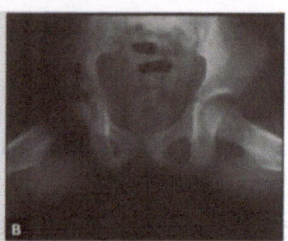

Figure 1. A, A patient aged 6 years with a Herring lateral pillar B Legg-Calvé-Perthes Disease of the hip in the reossification stage. B, Lateral radiographs showing Catteral Group IV disease. Because the patient is young, the prognosis is good.

Treatment

Nonsurgical

Treatment is not needed for patients with early disease who clinically have full, painless range of motion of the hip; on radiography are in Catterall group 1 or 2, Salter-Thompson Type A, or Herring lateral pillar Type A; have no head-at-risk signs. Patients with a painful, stiff hip should undergo home bed rest for 5 to 7 days and should take nonsteroidal anti-inflammatory drugs to control symptoms. Once the acute hip pain has resolved, gentle active and assisted passive range of motion of the hip is begun. Patients who do not respond to simple bed rest are hospitalized and placed in bilateral skin traction with progressive abduction over 7 to 10 days to mobilize the hip joint. Hips that do not regain full motion undergo arthrography; if lateral femoral head deformity is blocking hip abduction, no further containment treatment is possible. Hips that have an adduction contracture but are congruent on arthrography may benefit from percutaneous hip adductor release. Once maximum hip motion is obtained, containment therapy is considered for radiographic groups with poor prognosis. Although definitive proof of efficacy is lacking, the most widely used brace for hip containment is the Atlanta Scottish Rite hip abduction orthosis. This ambulatory brace holds the hip in abduction and slight flexion with external rotation, and it is well tolerated by children. It is worn an average of 6 to 18 months and can be discontinued when the head reaches the reossification stage. Bracing may also be considered for hips with Herring lateral pillar type B and hips prone to loss of motion.

Surgical

In patients who would qualify for brace treatment but are noncompliant, innominate pelvis osteotomy and hip varus osteotomy are used to contain the femoral head in the acetabulum. The hip joint must have full range of motion before surgery, it must be congruent, and the femoral head must be contained in a position of abduction and internal rotation. For the innominate osteotomy, the femoral head must also be spherical. Proponents of these procedures report results similar to those seen with bracing, but these treatments are costly and the complication rate is significant. Shelf arthroplasty has been advocated for children 8 years of age or older in Catterall groups 3 or 4. Patients with noncontainable hips and active disease or those with healed hips that have painful hinge abduction may benefit from an abduction-extension osteotomy of the hip. In skeletally mature patients, a cheilectomy may be considered.

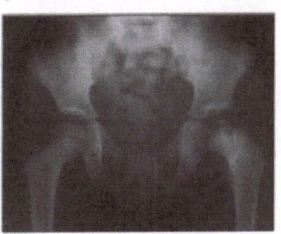

Figure 2. A lateral radiograph showing Catteral Group IV disease of the hip with whole head involvment in the fragmentation stage. Prognosis is guarded.

Key references
1. Catterall A: The natural history of Legg-Calvé-Perthes disease. *J Bone Joint Surg [Br]* 1971, 53:37.
2. Weinstein SL: Legg-Calvé-Perthes disease: results of long term follow-up. In *The Hip. Proceedings of the Thirteenth Open Scientific Meeting of the Hip Society.* Edited by Fitzgerald RH Jr. St. Louis: CV Mosby; 1985.
3. Yrjonen T: Prognosis in Perthes' disease after noncontainment treatment: 106 hips followed for 28–47 years. *Acta Orthop Scand* 1992, 63:523.

Diagnosis

History

Back pain ranks second only to upper respiratory illness as a reason for office visits to physicians and for loss of work. Eight of ten Americans will suffer from back pain at some time during their lives. A very careful history and physical examination are necessary. The exam should rule out other back problems that may be more serious and would require more urgent investigations and treatment. Patients should be asked about their history of back pain and any previous treatment or diagnostic modalities. The nature of the current pain and any exacerbating or relieving factors are important. Patients with chronic pain that worsens during time and is unrelated to activity should raise a suspicion of tumor. Important questions include whether the patient experiences nocturnal pain, involuntary weight loss, pain at rest, or if there is blood in the urine or stool. Patients can be divided into two groups: those with isolated low back pain and those with radicular symptoms into the lower extremities. Pain that radiates to the buttock and posterior thigh can result from pressure on the nerve supplying the annulus of a degenerative disk, osteoarthritis, or irritation of facet joints. Low back pain radiating past the knee into the calf or foot may reflect nerve compression which would be more commonly associated with a herniated disk, nerve compression from spinal osteophytes, or tumor.

Physical findings

Patients should be observed for their overall posture and gait patterns. Examine the patients' motor strength, reflexes, sensation to light touch and pin prick, lumbar spine range of motion, tension signs, and specific areas of tenderness. Percussion or palpation of the patient's spine will frequently exacerbate the pain. Flexion of the spine generally exacerbates the pain. Patients should be examined for toe walking and heel walking, which would identify gastrocnemius soleus (S1 radiculopathy) or ankle dorsiflexion (L5 radiculopathy) weakness, respectively. Nerve root tension tests (straight-leg raising, bow string test, femoral nerve stretch) are useful for assessing for nerve root compression. The straight-leg raise and bow string tests indicate L5 or S1 radiculopathies, which account for approximately 85% of disk herniations. Higher disk herniations at the L3 or L4 nerve roots may be detected with a positive femoral nerve stretch test. Motor examination can also help determine the level of nerve compression for an L4 lesion affecting the quadriceps, an L5 lesion affecting the great toe extensors and tibialis anterior muscle, or an S1 lesion affecting foot plantar flexion and peroneal muscles. Deep tendon reflexes should test the patellar (L3 and L4 nerve roots) and Achilles reflexes (S1 nerve root). Patients should be examined for inappropriate or "nonorganic" signs that correlate with psychologic distress. These signs are 1) superficial and widespread tenderness; 2) pain on axial loading of the spine (pressure on top of the head); 3) inconsistent pain on straight-leg raising in seated vs supine position, 4) regional disturbances of strength and sensation that do no correlate with dermatomal patterns, and 5) overreaction during the physical examination.

Imaging and laboratory studies

Anteroposterior and lateral radiographs of the lumbar spine are the initial studies. Any gross abnormalities such as degenerative changes, spondylolisthesis, blastic or lytic lesions, osteoporosis, or compression fractures may be diagnosed. Patients who have radicular symptoms may need further diagnostic work-ups, including magnetic resonance imaging, computed tomography, myelography, or electromyelographic testing. Radiographic studies are not needed in all patients with isolated back pain, because most cases of acute back pain resolve spontaneously within several weeks. Persistent pain or history of trauma necessitates radiographic studies. Flexion and extension lateral radiographs may show segmental instability with translation of one vertebral body on another.

Complications

Patients with low back pain or radicular symptoms have a large differential diagnosis. Failure to diagnose many of these conditions could result in severe progressive neurologic dysfunction and permanent deficits.

Differential diagnosis

Low back pain can arise from numerous structures in the lumbar spine including intervertebral ligaments, outer fibers of the annulus fibrosus, outer fibers, vertebral periosteum, paravertebral musculature, fascia, blood vessels, and nerve roots. These structures cause back pain by musculoligamentous injuries, degenerative changes of the intervertebral disks or facet joints, spinal stenosis, herniation of the nucleus pulposus (HNP), scoliosis, spondylolisthesis, primary or metastatic tumors, spinal infections, ankylosing spondylitis, peripheral vascular disease, aortic aneurysm, diseases of the pelvic organs, kidneys, or gastrointestinal tract, vertebral compression fractures, osteomalacia, Paget's disease of bone, or depression.

Etiology and pathophysiology

In most patients, low back pain is musculoskeletal in nature and caused by local injury to the intervertebral ligamentous structures or paraspinal musculature with inflammation and muscle spasms. In patients with lumbar degenerative disk disease, pain may result from local nerve compression. Pain may originate from the innervation of the annulus fibrosus or the facet joints. Local mediators of the pain have been identified, including substance P, prostaglandins, nitric oxide, IL-1, and IL-6.

Epidemiology

Approximately 70% to 80% of adults will have low back pain in their lives. Only 14% of adults have an episode that lasts more than 2 weeks. About 1.5% of such episodes will exhibit a sciatica-type pain. It has been estimated that 85% of patients with low back pain cannot be given a definitive diagnosis at the time of initial evaluation. The percentage of patients with low back pain who undergo surgery for disk herniation is approximately 2%. It is estimated that of all patients with low back pain, approximately 4% will have compression fractures, 3% spondylolisthesis, 0.7% spinal malignant neoplasms (primary or metastatic), 0.3% ankylosing spondylitis, and 0.01% spinal infections. The prevalence of HNP is complicated because 30% of asymptomatic patients under 40 years of age and 93% of asymptomatic patients over 60 years of age will have HNP on MRI.

Treatment

Nonsurgical

Patients without a spinal emergency can be treated conservatively. Treatment is directed specifically toward the etiology of the pain and most often consists of a combination therapies including nonsteroidal anti-inflammatory drugs, analgesics, muscle relaxants when indicated for muscle spasm, lumbar brace or corset (in cases of spinal instability), and application of heat to the lumbar spine. Physical therapy is beneficial for the overall range-of-motion and back strengthening exercises. Strengthening is directed at both the abdominal and paraspinal supporting musculature. Pelvic stabilization exercises are beneficial also. Aerobic conditioning, weight loss, and aquatic therapy are beneficial in most patients. Patients with radicular symptoms and evidence of nerve root compression may benefit from a short course of oral steroids or, in more severe cases, epidural steroid injections. Most patients with low back complaints improve within 1 to 2 weeks, regardless of the treatment. The key to successful long-term management of patients with low back pain may rely more on patient education and prevention of recurrent injury than on the acute initial management of the patient's symptoms.

Surgical

Patients with a spinal emergency like cauda equina syndrome require urgent surgical intervention for decompression of the neural elements. In patients with nerve compression secondary to a HNP, spondylolisthesis, and spinal stenosis, surgical intervention may be warranted because of failure of conservative treatment. Surgery may also be indicated for patients with demonstrated symptomatic lumbar instability as assessed on dynamic flexion-extension radiographs. Internal fixation with spinal instrumentation is necessary for patients with demonstrated instability or those undergoing arthrodesis (fusion) secondary to degenerative disorders. The results of arthrodesis for isolated low back pain secondary to degenerative disk disease are less satisfactory than results in patients undergoing decompression for compressed neural elements.

Exercise and activity modification

Patients with severe musculoskeletal back pain are encouraged to return rapidly to activity after taking a few days of rest. Back range-of-motion and strengthening exercises are initiated early. Physical therapy for education and progressive activity are vital. Avoidance of exacerbating factors (heavy lifting, bending, poor posture, stooping) also speed recovery.

Treatment aims

To restore patients to a full, active, asymptomatic productive lifestyle. Treatment is aimed at relieving the symptoms of initial pain and educating and rehabilitating patients in an attempt to prevent reinjury in the future. The goals of surgical treatment are to alleviate pain and prevent progressive neurologic injury in patients with compressed neural elements.

Prognosis

The prognosis for most patients with low back pain is excellent. Most patients will undergo complete recovery within 2 weeks, regardless of treatment prescribed. More than 90% of patients with an HNP will be managed successfully with nonoperative treatment, and in those who require surgical diskectomy, short-term studies have demonstrated a 90% to 95% success rate. Likewise, more than 70% of patients with symptomatic spondylolisthesis or spinal stenosis are managed successfully with conservative treatment. Patients who undergo surgical decompression or stabilization for more involved diseases (severe degenerative disorders) have a less favorable long-term prognosis. To rule out more serious pathology, patients with acute low back pain should be followed until symptoms subside. Failure to improve within the first 2 to 3 weeks should raise suspicion of a more serious pain etiology.

Key references

1. Deyo RA, Rainville J, Kent DL: What can the history and physical examination tell us about low back pain? *JAMA* 1992, 268:760–765.

2. Mooney V: Treating low back pain with exercise. *J Musculoskeletal Med* 1995, 12:24–36.

3. Saal JA, Saal JS: Nonoperative treatment of lumbar intervertebral discs with radiculopathy: an outcome study. *Spine* 1989, 14:431–437.

4. Waddel G, McCulloch JA, Kummel ED, et al.: Nonorganic physical signs and low back pain. *Spine* 1980, 5:117–125.

A. Agarwal

Diagnosis

History
Most patients present with a history of injury to the finger. This usually occurs during participation in a sporting event, especially basketball and baseball. Injury can also occur during an occupational or home activity. Patients most often report "jamming" the end of the finger on a baseball or basketball. After the injury, pain and inability to extend the involved finger develop. Occasionally, the injury can be caused by a laceration over the distal interphalangeal joint.

Physical findings
Patients present with swelling and inability to extend the distal interphalangeal joint of the injured finger. An associated laceration on the dorsum of the finger may be present. Neurovascular status is usually not compromised unless an associated laceration is present.

Imaging and laboratory studies
Plain radiographs of the finger (three views) are the diagnostic standard.

Complications
A major complication is the failure to diagnose and treat a mallet finger. This results in a chronic mallet finger and the need for an arthrodesis or secondary tendon reconstruction. Nonoperative treatment of these injuries is associated with a 45% rate of skin problems. Excessive hyperextension with a dorsal splint leads to full-thickness necrosis and nail deformities because of the pressure. Infection resulting from an open injury or after surgery is rare.

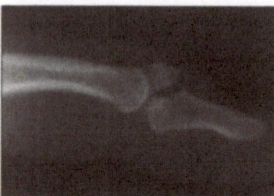

Figure 1. A Type IV(b) bony mallet finger.

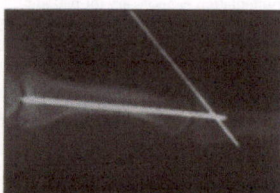

Figure 2. Treatment of mallet finger using Kirschner (K) wire fixation. The patient went on to solid union with full range of motion.

Differential diagnosis
Loss of extension can be caused by rupture of the tendon proximally and may be the result of trauma or systemic disorders, such as rheumatoid arthritis. Fractures of the distal phalanx or proximal phalanx can resemble a mallet finger. Severe arthritis of the distal interphalangeal joint can cause deformity of the joint and an inability to extend the finger.

Etiology or pathophysiology
Usual mechanism of injury is sudden acute forceful flexion of the extended finger at the distal interphalangeal joint. This causes rupture of the extensor tendon. There may be an associated small fragment of bone from its dorsal insertion onto the distal phalanx. Forced hyperextension of this same joint can also result in a mallet finger. This usually results in a much larger fracture of the distal phalanx that involves more than 30% of the joint. Rupture of the tendon at its terminal insertion may be related to the relative avascularity present in the area of the tendon overlying the joint. This would also explain the poor results associated with direct suturing of the ruptured tendon and the skin problems associated with splint treatment.

Epidemiology
Usually occurs in young male patients because it is frequently sports related. A classification scheme with some treatment implications has been proposed. A Type I injury (most common) is a closed injury caused by blunt trauma. There is loss of tendon continuity with or without a small avulsion fracture; Type II is a laceration at or just proximal to the distal interphalangeal joint with loss of tendon function; Type III injury involves a deep abrasion with loss of skin, subcutaneous tissue, and tendon substance; Type IV injury is subclassified into three categories: Type IV(a), a transepiphyseal plate fracture in children, Type IV(b), a hyperflexion injury with a fracture of 20% to 50% of the articular surface (Fig. 1), and Type IV(c), a hyperextension injury with a fracture involving more than 50% of the articular surface . Type IV(c) has volar subluxation of the distal phalanx. The mallet finger is also categorized as a zone I extensor tendon injury.

Treatment

Nonsurgical

A Type I injury is best treated by a dorsal or volar splint. Care should be taken to avoid excessive hyperextension, which may lead to complications. Types II and III mallet fingers are treated in a similar fashion after initial operative wound care.

Surgical

Types II and III injuries are best managed by urgent irrigation and debridement and care of the open wound. The mallet finger itself is best treated nonsurgically. Only Type IV injuries require true operative intervention, in the form of closed reduction and percutaneous pinning with 0.028 Kirschner (K) wires (Fig. 2). As an alternative, stainless steel figure eight wire, stainless steel pull-out wire, or pull-through sutures over a button can be used. The pull-through suture technique has been shown to be the most biomechanically stable construct. Surgery should be considered for injuries that are associated with significant joint involvement and demonstrate subluxation of the distal interphalangeal joint.

Exercise and activity modification

Protection of the finger from reinjury is the most important activity modification. The splint provides some protection. Sporting activities should be avoided when reinjury is a possibility.

Treatment aims
To reestablish the continuity of the extensor tendon and allow active extension at the distal interphalangeal joint. This goal should be met, and complications from splinting should be avoided.

Prognosis
If treated early, Type I mallet fingers have excellent result in 80% of cases. The 20% of cases with fair to poor results are due to a delay in diagnosis, delay in treatment, or improper splinting. The prognosis of the other types depends on the associated soft tissue injury (Types II and III) and the amount of articular damage (Type IV). Surgical treatment of these injuries is uniformly disappointing, although the best clinical results are with the pull-through suture technique.

Follow-up and management
All injuries are splinted for 6 weeks, followed by night splinting for 2 to 4 weeks. Active, active-assist, and passive range of motion can then be started at the end of the 6 weeks.

Key references
1. Damron TA, Engber WD: Surgical treatment of mallet finger fractures by tension band technique. *Clin Orthop* 1994, 300:133–139.
2. Damron TA, Engber WD, Lange RH, et al.: Biomechanical analysis of mallet finger fracture fixation techniques. *J Hand Surg* 1993, 18A:600–607.
3. Doyle JR: Extensor tendon injuries. In *Hand Surgery Update* vol I. Edited by Manske PR. American Academy of Orthopaedic Surgeons; 1996:149–160.

J.D. Heckman

Diagnosis

History

The patient reports flexion deformity of the distal interphalangeal joint of the toe, usually associated with pain over the tip of the toe (Fig. 1). Sometimes a painful callus develops over the tip of the toe because of excess pressure with walking.

Physical findings

A mallet toe is characterized by a flexion contracture of the distal interphalangeal joint of one of the lesser toes. Examination reveals a fixed-flexion deformity of the distal interphalangeal joint and, often, a tender callus on the tip of the toe. With a severe mallet toe deformity, the toenail may be deformed; an ingrown nail can result from repetitive pressure as it is driven into the ground with weight bearing.

Imaging and laboratory studies: anteroposterior and lateral radiographs of the digit show a flexion deformity of the distal interphalangeal joint.

Complications

A severe mallet toe can lead to ulceration of the tip of the toe, particularly in patients with loss of protective sensation, such as that caused by diabetes mellitus. An ingrown toenail can also result from the excessive pressure with weight bearing.

Differential diagnosis

A mallet toe deformity should be distinguished from a clawtoe deformity. The latter is more extensive, affecting the proximal joints of the digit as well.

Etiology or pathophysiology

Mallet toe results from a muscle imbalance in which the flexor digitorum longus overpowers the extensor digitorum longus, creating a fixed flexion deformity of the distal interphalangeal joint.

Epidemiology

Although this condition can be seen in such neuromuscular disorders as polio and cerebral palsy, it also occurs without any obvious underlying neurologic disease.

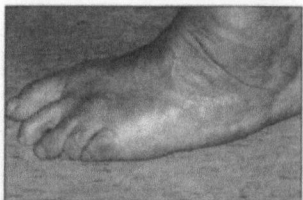

Figure 1. Second toe shows typical mallet deformity.

Treatment

Nonsurgical

Symptoms of mallet toe are aggravated by shoewear that is too tight. All efforts should be made to have the patient wear sensible shoes—ones with a wide and deep toe box. Usually, most of the symptoms are related to the painful callus on the tip of the toe. Pressure on the tip of the toe can be relieved by placing a metatarsal pad inside the shoe or placing a small pad under the proximal portion of the digit to keep the tip of the toe from touching the ground with weight bearing. A hypertrophic callus should be regularly sanded or trimmed to keep it from getting too large.

Surgical

Surgical treatment is designed to correct the flexion deformity of the distal interphalangeal joint. Often, the only procedure required is a simple surgical transection of the flexor digitorum longus tendon, just proximal to its insertion on the base of the distal phalanx. Sometimes, however, the soft tissues are contracted and a flexor tendon release alone will not correct the deformity. In such cases, the contracted joint capsule must also be released. When the toenail has become deformed or ulceration on the tip of the toe recurs, a terminal Syme's amputation should be seriously considered. In this procedure, the toenail and its matrix, along with the distal phalanx of the digit, are resected to correct the deformity. A second surgical technique involves resection arthroplasty or arthrodesis of the distal interphalangeal joint. With both of these techniques, the deformity is corrected and the distal phalanx is aligned with the middle phalanx. With resection arthroplasty, scar tissue fills the defect and holds the tip of the toe straight; with fusion, an actual bony bridge maintains correction of the deformity for the long term.

Treatment aims
To relieve pain and prevent callus build-up and chronic ulceration of the tip of the toe.

Prognosis
The prognosis for mallet toe is generally good. It usually responds to nonsurgical treatment, but fixed deformities may need to be corrected surgically. Surgical release of the flexor tendon or amputation of the tip of the toe usually relieves the patient's symptoms in both the short and long term.

Follow-up and management
Even after surgical correction the patients should be encouraged to wear sensible shoes with a wide, deep toe box that will accommodate the affected toe as well as the adjacent toes.

Key references
1. Coughlin MJ: Operative repair of the mallet toe deformity. *Foot Ankle Int* 1995, 16:109–116.

R.C. Schenck, Jr.

Diagnosis

History

Sprain of the medial collateral ligament (MCL) of the knee is the most common ligamentous injury to the knee. It usually results from a twisting injury in which the foot remains fixed (eg, when a patient falls while skiing and the boot does not release from the ski, causing a twisting injury) or from a lateral sided blow from a fall or sporting injury. Acute pain and medial-sided knee swelling occur, with eventual ecchymosis medially. After the injury, weight bearing and knee motion (especially extension) are difficult because of pain.

Physical findings

The acute MCL sprain is accompanied by medial knee swelling with limited active range of motion secondary to pain. Ecchymosis and tenderness may be present along the MCL. Careful palpation is required to identify the injured structure; knowledge of the underlying anatomy is necessary to make the clinical correlation of anatomy to the injured structure. With mild sprains, tenderness is usually in the area of the medial femoral epicondyle (ligament origin); with severe sprains, the tenderness is usually diffuse along the MCL and frequently occurs along the tibial insertion 2 to 4 cm distal to the joint line. Grading of the MCL injury is in accordance with American Medical Association guidelines for ligament sprains. Grade I implies microscopic tearing, grade II implies macroscopic tearing, and grade III implies complete injury. Valgus stress testing with the knee in slight flexion (20°) and comparison to the normal contralateral knee is graded by joint line opening (0- to 5-mm opening, grade I; 5- to 10-mm opening, grade II; greater than 10-mm opening, grade III) (Fig. 1). Integrity of the anterior cruciate ligament (ACL) is imperative for proper management of the MCL. The integrity of the ACL is best evaluated with a careful Lachman examination.

Imaging and laboratory studies

Plain radiographs are necessary to rule out fracture (lateral plateau fracture could create abnormal findings on valgus examination because of fracture displacement). The patient should be carefully evaluated for epicondylar fracture fragments or evidence of a Segond's fracture (implying cruciate tear). Magnetic resonance imaging can be used to grade the MCL injury but is no substitute for clinical examination. However, this imaging test is useful for evaluation of associated injuries, such as meniscal or ACL tears.

Complications

Complications from an MCL injury stem from an inaccurate diagnosis. Careful evaluation for fracture or an associated ACL tear is key to successful management.

Differential diagnosis

With valgus instability, fracture of the knee or injury to one of the cruciate ligaments can occur. Clinicians discuss "isolating" the diagnosis of the MCL—that is, ruling out other injuries. Presence of a concomitant ACL tear (ie, ACL/MCL tears) completely changes the management and overall outcome of such a knee injury.

Etiology or pathophysiology

Sprains of the MCL occur secondary to a valgus blow to the lateral aspect of the knee or with an external rotation force placed on the tibia. These injuries are traumatic in origin.

Epidemiology

Sprains of the MCL occur in adults and are associated with sporting activities and injuries.

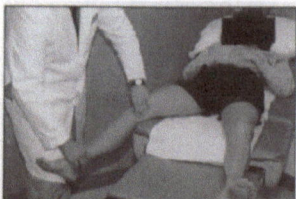

Figure 1. A doctor performs a valgus stress test.

Treatment

Nonsurgical

Nonsurgical treatment is based on the integrity of the ACL. With isolated MCL sprains, meniscal tears are rare and can also be ruled out with magnetic resonance imaging. The severity or grade of sprain is a reliable predictor of the time to return to activity and duration of short-term disability. Treatment of the acute MCL sprain involves short-term joint rest; icing; and, within 48 hours, the institution of a rehabilitation program that includes range-of-motion exercises and weight bearing as tolerated. Grade I and grade II MCL sprains respond quickly to such management and have been shown to recover fully in 3 to 10 days (grade I) to 1 to 3 weeks (grade II). Grade III sprains are frequently treated by use of a brace for range-of-motion exercises; patients can usually return to activities in 3 to 6 weeks. Thigh musculature strengthening and weight-bearing exercises can promote maintenance of knee function and prevent quadriceps atrophy.

Surgical

There is no indication for surgical treatment of an acute isolated MCL sprain, regardless of the injury. With an intact ACL, the MCL has an "internal" collateral (or splint) that allows it to heal without surgery. Clinical trials that have studied surgical repair of complete (grade III) MCL tears have shown that patients who underwent surgery had increased complications (stiffness) compared with patients managed without surgery.

Exercise and activity modification

For the short term, patients should avoid running or cutting activities to allow adequate ligament healing.

Treatment aims
To allow ligamentous healing and quick restoration of function.

Prognosis
The prognosis for grade I and grade II MCL sprains is excellent. Grade III isolated MCL tears also heal nonoperatively with routinely good results. However, in a small percentage of patients (<10%) with grade III MCL sprains or valgus—especially athletes in positions that entail high-level skill—instability can occur. In such patients, the use of bracing during strenuous activities is advised.

Rehabilitation
A functional sports-specific rehabilitation program is used, with a focus on quadriceps strength and weight-bearing activities. Early gait training is frequently required to avoid a limp; although simplistic, this training hastens the time to recovery. Quadriceps strengthening is performed with closed chain (weight bearing—ie, partial squats to 30°) exercises. Straight-leg-raise strengthening should be performed with the leg in internal rotation to avoid stretching of the healing MCL secondary to gravity.

Key references

1. Felto JF, Marsine JL: Medial collateral ligament injuries of the knee: a rationale for treatment. *Clin Orthop* 1978, 132:206.

2. Indelicato PA, Hermarsdorfer J, Huegel M: Nonoperative management of complete tears of the medial collateral ligament of the knee in intercollegiate football players. *Clin Orthop* 1990, 256:174–177.

Diagnosis

History

Most patients who present with metacarpal fractures report being involved in some altercation. The event often entails punching either a wall or a person. Fractures of the metacarpal can result from any type of trauma, however, including motor vehicle collisions and crush injuries.

Physical findings

Physical examination reveals swelling over the dorsum of the hand. There is pain on palpation, and the involved finger may have a rotational deformity. Pain may also prevent the patient from flexing the finger. It is important to look for an associated open wound, which may indicate a "fight bite." Nerve and vascular injuries are rare, occurring only when the mechanism involves a severe crush injury with associated soft tissue loss.

Imaging and laboratory studies

Plain radiographs of the hand (Fig.1) are sufficient for evaluation of metacarpal fractures.

Complications

Complications occur with both surgical and nonsurgical treatment. Surgical complications include tendon adherence with resultant limitation of motion. This may require surgical tenolysis if motion is severely limited. Malunion and joint stiffness occur more frequently after nonsurgical treatment (Fig. 2). Severe malunion, which is usually rotational in nature, can require osteotomy and plating for correction of the deformity. Nonunion can occur after either type of treatment but fortunately is rare.

Differential diagnosis

A simple soft tissue contusion or a shooter's abscess can cause swelling on the dorsum of the hand. Plain films and clinical history will help in the diagnosis. Carpometacarpal fracture-dislocations can also present in a similar fashion.

Etiology or pathophysiology

The mechanism of injury is directly due to bending forces that occur with axial loading of the metacarpal. This results in a transverse fracture of the shaft. Torsional loading causes a spiral or oblique fracture. An example of axial loading occurs when a wall is hit while the fist is clenched. This usually results in a "boxer's fracture." Metacarpal fractures can result from direct trauma to the hand; such injuries tend to cause comminuted fractures.

Epidemiology

Metacarpal fractures account for approximately 36% of all hand fractures. Of all these, the boxer's fracture, a fifth metacarpal neck fracture, accounts for 20%. Young male patients are more frequently affected because of the traumatic nature of the injury. Metacarpal fractures may be transverse, spiral, oblique, or comminuted.

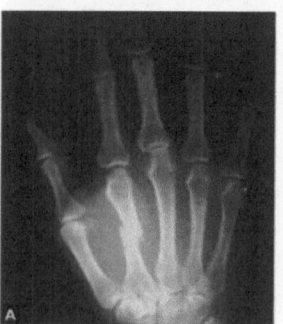

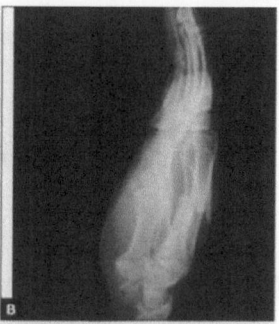

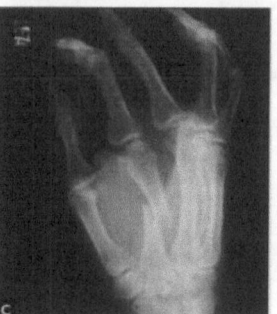

Figure 1. A, Anteroposterior (AP), B, lateral, and C, oblique views of a shaft fracture of the second metacarpus.

Treatment

Nonsurgical

Almost all boxer's fractures can be treated with closed reduction and an ulnar gutter splint. Some authors have advocated buddy taping with early motion. Up to 70° of angular deformity can be accepted without functional loss. As a result, this injury is extremely amenable to nonoperative management. Diaphyseal fractures of the metacarpal shaft can be treated with splint or cast immobilization as long as no rotational or angular deformity is present. If an attempt at closed reduction does not resolve the malalignment, surgical intervention should be considered. The metacarpal can also become shortened, especially with spiral or oblique patterns; this makes restoration of length difficult without an outrigger apparatus. Transverse fractures of the metacarpal are unstable and often require surgery. Closed reduction of these fractures can be successful, however, with proper casting and reduction techniques.

Surgical

Surgical intervention should be considered for certain situations only. Nonoperative treatment can be tried initially for all closed injuries. However, the failure to obtain and maintain satisfactory alignment after closed reduction warrants surgical treatment. Any open fracture, including associated fractures of the fifth metacarpal neck ("fight bites"), is a surgical emergency. These fractures require irrigation and debridement in the operating room, with or without stabilization. Displaced intra-articular fractures require anatomic reduction of the joint surface to minimize future arthritic changes. If multiple fractures or a significant soft tissue injury is present, surgical stabilization with pins or plates and screws should be considered.

Exercise and activity modification

Exercise and activity are restricted during the healing of these fractures because the patient is usually immobilized. Surgical treatment of these fractures with open reduction and internal fixation allows early motion, but participation in activities will be limited until healing has occurred.

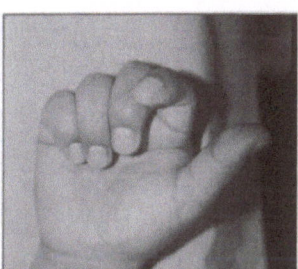

Figure 2. A clinical photograph of the resultant malrotation of the healed metacarpal shaft fracture.

Treatment aims
To prevent deformity of the hand and finger during the healing process. In surgical treatment, the goal is to provide anatomic reduction with stable fixation that allows early active motion.

Prognosis
Overall, prognosis is excellent. Surgical treatment results in excellent clinical results in more than 90% of cases.

Follow-up and management
Nonsurgical treatment of metacarpal fractures in a splint or cast is maintained for 4 to 6 weeks depending on radiographic and clinical findings of healing. Treatment with open reduction and internal fixation allows early active motion after only 2 to 3 weeks of splinting. All fractures should be followed until the fracture heals and normal hand function returns.

Key references
1. Ashkenaze DM, Ruby L: Metacarpal fractures and dislocations. *Orthop Clin North Am* 1992, 23:19–33.
2. Bosscha K, Snellen JP: Internal fixation of metacarpal and phalangeal fractures with AO minifragment screws and plates: a prospective study. *Injury* 1993, 24:166–168.

P.L.J. McGanity

Diagnosis

History
Most metatarsal fractures commonly result from direct insult to the forefoot. Less common mechanisms of injury include indirect torsional force to the forefoot and avulsion injury to the proximal metatarsal base.

Physical findings
Pain over the dorsum of the forefoot that increases with weight bearing or dependency.

Point tenderness with palpation at the fracture site occurring soon after injury.

Axial or torsional force applied to the toe or toes causing pain at the fracture.

Swelling and bruising of the forefoot.

Imaging and laboratory studies
Three radiographic views of the foot should be obtained: anteroposterior, lateral, and oblique. The anteroposterior and oblique views more commonly demonstrate the fracture and its pattern. The lateral view is most important for determination of plantar or dorsal fracture displacement.

Complications
Failure to recognize significant plantar or dorsal fracture displacement may lead to fracture malunion. Plantar malunion may cause pain with weight bearing or plantar callus formation. Dorsal malunion may cause pain with shoe wearing if a low toe box rubs on the foot.

Differential diagnosis
Injury to the base of the toe, Lisfranc midfoot injury, and forefoot compartment syndrome should be considered during evaluation of forefoot trauma.

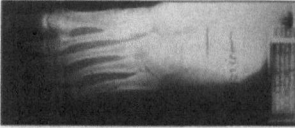

Figure 1. Radiograph of a metatarsal fracture.

Treatment

Nonsurgical

The workhorse of treatment is nonsurgical. Early weight bearing as symptoms allow is important in preventing stiffness and decreasing the need for pain medication. Weight bearing also reduces the period of patient disability.

Surgical

Surgery is rarely indicated. The most common indications are significant frontal displacement of fractures of the first or fifth metatarsal and significant sagittal displacement of any metatarsal.

Treatment aims
To achieve a painless, fully functional foot within 100 days of injury.
To allow use of regular shoes for normal walking in that same period.

Prognosis
Prognosis is excellent when the forefoot has not been crushed. When a crush injury has caused the fracture, prognosis is more guarded because of the severity of soft tissue damage.

Follow-up and management
Early follow-up of proximal metatarsal fractures, especially the second metatarsal, is important so that a more serious Lisfranc injury is not overlooked. Weight bearing should be encouraged soon after simple fractures to prevent forefoot stiffness and reduce postinjury edema. Active and passive toe motion helps accelerate recovery.

Key references
1. Dameron TB: Fractures and anatomical variations of the proximal portion of the fifth metatarsal. *J Bone Joint Surg* 1975, 57A:788–792.
2. Heckman JD: Fractures and dislocations of the foot. In *Rockwood and Green's Fractures in Adults* edn 4. Philadelphia: Lippincott Williams and Wilkins; 1996:2373–2382.
3. Shereff MJ: Fractures of the forefoot. *Instructional Course Lectures.* Rosemont, IL: American Academy of Orthopaedic Surgeons; 1990:133–140.

Diagnosis

History

Patients with metatarsalgia report pain in the forefoot that is usually aggravated by standing and walking. The pain may range from aching and throbbing to burning sensations. It is commonly aggravated by tight shoewear and may be more prominent with vigorous athletic activities such as running and jumping. Metatarsalgia is not a specific disease but rather a symptom complex with many different causes.

Physical findings

The physical findings vary depending on the specific cause of the metatarsalgia. One of the most common causes is a painful callus or corn. Calluses develop on the plantar aspect of the foot under one or more metatarsal heads. The callus becomes thickened with weight bearing and then becomes more painful. Painful soft corns can develop in the web spaces between the toes, particularly between the fourth and fifth toes. Careful inspection of the web space will identify these hyperkeratotic lesions. Other conditions that can cause metatarsalgia are arthritis of the metatarsophalangeal joints, rheumatoid arthritis, stress fracture of a metatarsal, Morton's interdigital neuroma, bunion, and bunionette.

Imaging and laboratory studies

Standing anteroposterior lateral and oblique radiographs of the foot should be obtained to identify any underlying bony abnormality, such as arthritis of the metatarsophalangeal joints and stress fracture of the metatarsal shaft. Diagnostic 1% Xylocaine injections can be helpful in differentiating the causes of metatarsalgia. Xylocaine injection of a Morton's interdigital neuroma or an arthritic joint should substantially relieve symptoms.

Complications

Serious systemic diseases, such as rheumatoid arthritis or a painful bone tumor, are sometimes the cause of metatarsalgia. Careful inspection of the radiographs will usually identify these more serious disorders.

Differential diagnosis

Among the many causes of metatarsalgia are plantar calluses, interdigital soft corns, arthritis of the metatarsophalangeal joints, stress fracture of the metatarsal shaft, and Morton's interdigital neuroma.

Etiology or pathophysiology

Most of the causes of metatarsalgia are precipitated by excessive weight-bearing activities and too-tight shoewear. Judicious use of appropriate shoewear and limitation of physical activities often controls symptoms.

Epidemiology

Metatarsalgia remains one of the more common musculoskeletal symptom complexes.

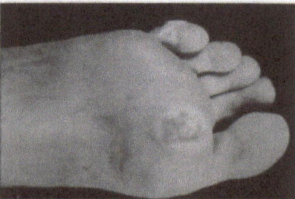

Figure 1. A common cause of metatarsalgia is a thick callus underlying the second metatarsal head.

Treatment

Nonsurgical

Because most causes of metatarsalgia are aggravated by shoewear and excessive weight-bearing activities, the first management step should always be shoewear modification. The toe box of the shoe should be wide enough and deep enough to accommodate the toes. This goal can usually be accomplished with an Oxford-type shoe. When the cause of the metatarsalgia is a painful plantar callus or a Morton's neuroma, a metatarsal pad placed judiciously in the shoe, lying just proximal to the metatarsal heads, often relieves the weight-bearing pressure on the metatarsal heads, relieving the patient's symptoms. Donut-type foam rubber pads placed around painful bony prominences also relieve shoe pressure.

Surgical

Surgical treatment should be reserved for conditions that do not respond to nonsurgical treatment. The specific surgical treatments should be directed at the underlying abnormality. A chronically inflamed Morton's neuroma can be excised. Arthritic joints can be treated either by resection arthroplasty or arthrodesis, and painful corns can be treated by resection of the underlying bony prominences. Only rarely is surgical treatment needed to treat a painful plantar callus.

Exercise and activity modification

Shoewear modification should be combined with activity modification when possible. Prolonged standing and walking often aggravate metatarsalgia. Patients should participate in fitness activities that do not apply repetitive loading stresses to the foot; such activities as cycling and swimming are most compatible with a healthy lifestyle while minimizing stress applied to the forefoot.

Treatment aims
To relieve painful forefoot symptoms.

Prognosis
The prognosis for metatarsalgia is generally good. After a vigorous diagnostic effort is made to clearly define the cause of the forefoot pain, treatment can be directed specifically at its management.

Follow-up and management
Metatarsalgia can recur if a long-term solution to the problem is not found. Often the use of modified shoewear and modification of athletic and work activities must persist indefinitely in order to continue to control the symptoms.

Key references
1. Gould JS: Metatarsalgia. Orthop Clin North Am 1989, 25:53–62.
2. Trnka HJ, Muhlbauer M, Zett LR, et al.: Comparison of the results of the Werl and Helao osteotomies for the treatment of metatarsalgia secondary to dislocation of the lesser metatarsophalangeal joints. Foot Ankle Int 1999, 20:72–79.

J.R. Warman

Diagnosis

History
Forefoot adduction is present from birth. No symptoms are typically noted. If, however, a rigid metatarsus adductus is not corrected during infancy, difficulty and pain with shoewear may occur.

Physical findings
The forefoot is adducted compared with the hindfoot (Fig. 1). The foot can be supple and easily passively corrected past neutral or can be more rigid and not correctable. Ankle and subtalar motion are normal.

Imaging and laboratory studies
Radiographs: usually unnecessary. Radiographic views will show the adduction of the forefoot at the tarsometatarsal joints.

Complications
The incidence of developmental hip dysplasia may be increased in infants with metatarsus adductus.

Differential diagnosis
Do not confuse with a clubfoot. Metatarsus adductus is one component of a clubfoot deformity, which also consists of hindfoot varus and ankle equinus.

Etiology or pathophysiology
No cause has been proven, but the condition is believed to be secondary to intrauterine positioning.

Epidemiology
The incidence is 1 per 1000 births.

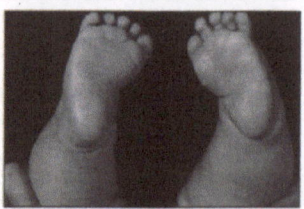

Figure 1. Forefoot adduction in metatarsus adductus.

Treatment

Nonsurgical

If the deformity is mild, the clinician need only reassure the parents. If the foot is stiff and cannot be corrected past neutral serial casting is indicated. Children younger than 1 year will have the best results. Casts are applied weekly until correction is achieved; a holding cast is then placed for 2 weeks. Correction is maintained with a Denis-Browne bar with straight-last shoes during nighttime and naps for several months and straight-last shoes for daytime wear.

Surgical

Older children (past walking age) with stiff metatarsus adductus may need surgical correction. This can be achieved with multiple metatarsal osteotomies or a lateral column shortening, possibly combined with a medial column lengthening. An example is cuboid decancellation with or without placement of bone graft to lengthen the medial cuneiform.

Treatment aims

To achieve a supple forefoot that presents with no shoewear problems.

Prognosis

Passively correctable feet have an excellent result without treatment. Intervention is needed for moderate and severe deformities.

Follow-up and management

Any recurrence can be corrected with a second serial casting.

Key references

1. Sullivan JA: The child's foot. In *Lovell and Winter's Pediatric Orthopedics*. Edited by Morrissy RT, Weinstein SL. Philadelphia: Lippincott–Raven; 1996:1077–1083.

2. Thompson GH, Simons GW: Congenital talipes equinovarus (clubfeet) and metatarsus adductus. In *The Child's Foot*. Edited by Drennan JC. New York: Raven Press; 1992:123–128.

Diagnosis

History

Patients with Morton's interdigital neuroma present with chronic and persistent burning pain in the forefoot. The pain is often localized in the second or third web space but sometimes is diffuse and poorly localized. The pain is aggravated by standing and walking, particularly in tight shoewear. Pain is relieved only by sitting down, removing the shoe, and rubbing the forefoot. Patients sometimes report numbness in the affected web space.

Physical findings

Tenderness can often be localized to the affected web space, especially plantarly just at or distal to the level of the metatarsal heads. Manual medial–lateral compression of the metatarsal heads may also reproduce the discomfort and can produce a clicking sensation. The web space may have decreased sensation to light touch or pin prick. Splaying of the two toes may directly result from pressure of the neuroma, causing the digits to separate.

Imaging and laboratory studies

Radiographs of the forefoot are normal in this condition. One of the best ways to confirm the diagnosis is to inject 2 to 3 mL of 1% plain Xylocaine into the affected web space. The local block of the affected common digital nerve usually leads to complete, but transient, symptom relief.

Differential diagnosis

Morton's interdigital neuroma is one of the causes of metatarsalgia. Other conditions that should be considered in the differential diagnosis are painful corns and calluses, particularly a painful callus underlying one of the adjacent metatarsal heads. Pain in the web space can also be caused by arthritic changes in one of the adjacent metatarsophalangeal joints. The joints should be carefully examined through passive range of motion and axial loading to elicit any pain or crepitus indicative of degenerative changes or synovitis in the joint. A stress fracture of the metatarsal shaft can also cause pain to radiate out into the web space and confuse the diagnosis.

Etiology or pathophysiology

Morton's interdigital neuroma is caused by irritation of the common digital nerve as it passes across the firm transverse metatarsal ligament that bridges the metatarsal heads in the web space. Particularly with the use of high-heeled shoes, the common digital nerve can be "bow-strung" across the transverse metatarsal ligament, causing irritation and swelling of the nerve. As the nerve becomes swollen and inflamed, it is more easily irritated as it rides over the ligament; this, in turn, creates more swelling and eventually causes the formation of scar tissue in and around the nerve.

Epidemiology

This condition occurs commonly in adults, especially those who wear high-heeled, pointed-toed shoes and boots.

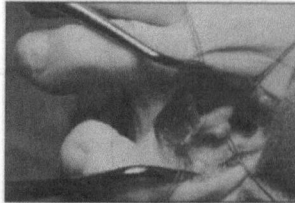

Figure 1. A typical Morton's interdigital neuroma. Surgical dissection shows thickened and inflammed common digital nerve.

Treatment

Nonsurgical
If a diagnostic injection with Xylocaine relieves the patient's symptoms, long-lasting relief can sometimes be obtained by injection of a local steroid preparation such as Celestone Soluspan (Schering, Kenilworth, NJ) injectable suspension. The bow-stringing effect of the transverse metatarsal ligament can also be minimized by placing a metatarsal pad in the patient's shoe just proximal to the level of the metatarsal heads. This pad decreases dorsiflexion at the metatarsophalangeal joints and decreases irritation of the common digital nerve. Patients should avoid wearing high-heeled, pointed-toed shoes as much as possible.

Surgical
Surgical treatment should be considered only when conservative treatment fails. The chronically inflamed and swollen nerve should be approached through a dorsal surgical incision in the web space. Transection of the transverse metatarsal ligament exposes the swollen and inflamed common digital nerve (the Morton's interdigital neuroma) in its entirety. Most authors recommend excision of the common digital nerve with resection of its contributing branches well proximal to the level of the transverse metatarsal ligament. Other authors simply recommend surgical transection of the transverse metatarsal ligament, alleviating the source of nerve irritation.

Exercise and activity modification
Patients with a symptomatic Morton's interdigital neuroma should avoid wearing high-heeled, pointed-toed shoes. Instead, they should wear shoes with an adequately-sized toe box.

Treatment aims
To relieve the pain of the inflamed common digital nerve.

Prognosis
The prognosis for recovery is generally good, and most patients respond to nonsurgical treatment. Surgical resection of the Morton's interdigital neuroma is effective in 90% to 95% of cases. In 5% to 10% of cases, the neuroma recurs, requiring further, more aggressive, and more extensive surgical treatment.

Follow-up and management
Recovery after surgical treatment is fairly rapid. The foot should be protected in a wooden-soled shoe for 3 to 4 weeks after surgery until the soft tissues have had a chance to heal. A vigorous range of motion exercise program for the toes should then be instituted to minimize stiffness and restore mobility.

Key references
1. Weinfeld SB, Myerson MS: Interdigital neuritis: diagnosis and treatment. *J Am Acad Orthop Surg* 1996, 4:328–335.

Pharmacology

Overview

Aspirin is the prototype of the nonsteroidal anti-inflammatory drugs (NSAIDs), which reduce but do not completely eliminate the signs and symptoms of established inflammation. This drug class has no major effect on the underlying disease process. Except for nabumetone, NSAIDs are organic acids that are highly bound to plasma proteins, a property that enhances their concentration in inflamed tissues.

COX-1 vs. COX-2 inhibitors

The NSAIDs inhibit cyclooxygenase (COX), the enzyme that transforms arachidonic acid into prostaglandins, prostacyclin, and thromboxanes. Recent work has focused on drugs that differentiate between inhibiting two different COXs: COX-1 inhibition, which is neither analgesic nor anti-inflammatory but does lead to gastric ulcers, and COX-2 inhibition, which spares the gastric mucosa but is both analgesic and anti-inflammatory (*eg*, celecoxib).

Adverse Effects

Gastrointestinal: gastric irritation and exacerbation of peptic ulcers. Celecoxib, a new COX-2 inhibitor, has minimal effects on the gastric mucosa.

Anticoagulant: decreased platelet adhesiveness, especially when exposed to aspirin. Displacement of warfarin from protein plasma protein-binding sites

Hepatic: reversible hepatocellular toxicity, characterized by elevations of one or more liver enzymes, may occur in up to 15% of patients receiving NSAIDs.

Renal: the NSAIDs may decrease creatinine clearance in some patients who are predisposed by hypovolemia, impaired renal function, or deceased renal blood flow.

Drug interactions: the NSAIDs may potentiate the effects of oral hypoglycemic agents and warfarin.

COX-2 inhibitors

Celecoxib (Celebrex; GD Searle & Co, Chicago, IL) and rofecoxib (Vioxx; Merck & Co, West Point, PA) are just two of the new COX-2 inhibitors that avoid many of the side effects of NSAIDs by targeting only the COX-2 enzyme.

Protective agents: misoprostol (Cytotec; GD Searle & Co, Chicago, IL)—100 to 200 µg four times a day protects both the stomach and the duodenum; ranitidine (Zantac; Glaxo Wellcome, Research Triangle Park, NC)—150 mg twice a day protection against duodenal ulcer formation.

Alternative NSAIDs: salsalate (Disalcid; 3M Pharmaceuticals, St. Paul, MN)—nonacetylated; nabumetone (Relafen; Smithkline Beecham Pharmaceuticals, Philadelphia, PA)—nonacidic; etodolac (Lodine; Wyeth-Ayerst Laboratories, Philadelphia, PA)—pyranocarboxylic acid.

NSAIDs and dosages

Drug	Trade Name	Dosage Range, mg/d	Pharmacologic Half-life, h	Doses Per Day	Gastrointestinal Adverse Effects*
Aspirin	Multiple trade names	1000–6000	4–15	2–4	+++
Celecoxib	Celebrex[†]	200–400	11	1–2	+
Diclofenac	Arthotec[†]	75–150	1–2	2–3	++
Diflunisal	Dolobid[‡]	500–1500	7–15	2	+++
Etodolac	Lodine[§]	600–1200	7	3–4	+
Flurbiprofen	Ansaid[¶]	100–300	3–4	2–3	++
Ibuprofen	Motrin[**]	1200–3200	2	3–6	++
Indomethacin	Indocine[‡]	50–200	3–11	2–4	+++
Ketoprofen	Orudis[§]	100–400	2	3–4	++
Ketorolac	Toradol[††]	15–150	4–6	4	+++
Nabumetone	Relafen[‡‡]	1000–2000	3–4	1–2	+
Naproxen	Naprosyn,[††] Aleve,[§§] Naprelan,[§]	250–1500	13–15	1–2	++
Oxaprozin	Daypro[†]	600–1200	21–25	1	+
Piroxicam	Feldene[¶¶]	20	30–86	1	+++
Salsalate	Disalcid[***]	1500–5000	4–15	2–4	+
Sulindac	Clinoril[‡]	300–400	16	2	+++
Tometin	Tolectin DS[**]	800–1600	1	4–6	+

*+ = none to mild, no change in drug regimen required; ++ = frequent, may need gastroprotective agent; +++ = more frequent or severe, often requires withdrawal of drug.
[†]GD Searle & Co, Chicago, IL.
[‡]Merck & Co, West Point, PA.
[§]Wyeth-Ayerst, Philadelphia, PA.
[¶]Pharmacia & Upjohn, Kalamazoo, MI.
[**]Ortho McNeil, Raritan, NJ.
[††]Syntex Laboratories, Palo Alto, CA.
[‡‡]SmithKline Beecham Pharmaceuticals, Philadelphia, PA.
[§§]Procter & Gamble Pharmaceuticals, Norwich, NY.
[¶¶]Pfizer, New York, NY.
[***]3M Pharmaceuticals, St. Paul, MN.

Key references

1. Snider RK: *Essentials of Musculoskeletal Care.* Rosemont, IL: American Academy of Orthopaedic Surgeons; 1997.

2. Schumacher HR: *Primer on Rheumatic Diseases* edn 10. Atlanta: The Arthritis Foundation; 1993.

Diagnosis

History

Nuresmaid's elbow is the clinical syndrome of painful limitation of motion of the elbow after traumatic interposition of the annular ligament into the radio-capitellar joint. The patient usually has a history of an abrupt pull on the upper extremity with sudden onset of pain and will not use the affected extremity. The classic scenario is of the "nursemaid" walking an unwilling toddler across the street, holding his hand; the child suddenly stops or drops to play, provoking a longitudinal traction injury to the arm. The injury can also occur during play with other children and with solitary falls.

Physical findings

The injured elbow is carried in flexion with the forearm pronated. The child is usually comfortable with this position but is in obvious distress with attempts to passively supinate the forearm. Tenderness over the radial head is always present. Passive flexion and extension of the elbow are usually painless.

Imaging and laboratory studies

An anteroposterior and lateral radiograph of the injured elbow is taken more to rule out fracture rather than to confirm nursemaid's elbow because with the latter, radiographs are normal. The definitive treatment of most nursemaid's elbows usually occurs when the x-ray technician supinates the forearm to obtain the anteroposterior view, with inadvertent reduction of the ligament.

Complications

No complications of nursemaid's elbow seem to occur when the elbow is reduced promptly, but untreated nursemaid's elbow may eventually require surgical removal of the interposed ligament to restore motion.

Differential diagnosis

Supracondylar fracture of the distal humerus.

Septic arthritis of the elbow.

Lateral condyle fracture of the distal humerus.

Elbow dislocation.

Etiology

The radial head in children is slightly oval, and cadaver studies in children younger that 5 years of age show that a traction injury to the elbow causes a distal tear of the annular ligament, allowing it to retract proximally into the radiocapitellar joint. In children older than 5 years, the same mechanism of injury could not produce a nursemaid's elbow; with increased force, however, full elbow dislocation occurred without tear of the annular ligament.

Epidemiology

Nursemaid's elbow has a peak incidence between 1 and 3 years of age but can be seen in children up to 5 years of age. It is a common injury of childhood, seen more often than fracture of the clavicle in children within the at-risk ages. The injury is more commonly seen in boys and most often involves the left elbow.

Treatment

While the elbow is held with a finger over the radial head, the other hand supinates the elbow; with successful reduction, a click is felt over the radial head (Fig. 1). The child may have instantaneous pain relief and return of full active motion of the elbow; in other children, several hours may be needed before symptoms resolve. Use of an overnight posterior elbow splint with an arm sling is helpful in some children. If reduction was successful, by the next day children should be asymptomatic and have full active use of the extremity.

When the simple supination maneuver cannot reduce the acute nursemaid's elbow, reduction may be obtained by both supinating the forearm and flexing the elbow. In the rare child with a persistently painful elbow despite reduction maneuvers, open surgical release of the interposed ligament may be indicated if elbow arthrography confirms the diagnosis.

Treatment aims

To exclude other causes of swollen, painful elbow mimicking nursemaid's elbow such as fracture.

To recognize and reduce a nursemaid's elbow in a timely fashion.

Prognosis

Most children with nursemaid's elbow are briefly symptomatic and spontaneously reduce the injury without treatment through elbow motion during play activities. Children who require manipulative reduction have a 5% risk for recurrence. Repeated reduction maneuvers are usually effective in these cases.

Follow-up and management

A follow-up telephone call to the family the day after the visit to determine whether the child is using the extremity normally is important. Children with persistent pain or limitation of elbow motion should be seen in the office for re-evaluation.

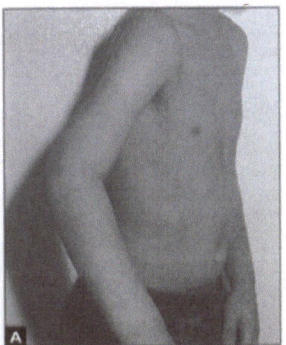
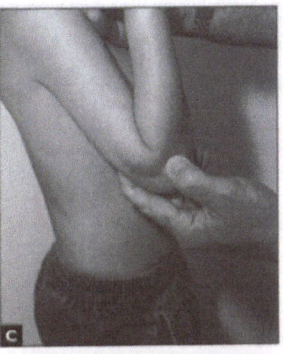
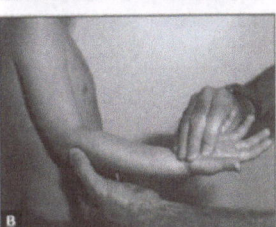

Figure 1. A, In nursemaid's elbow, the forearm is held in mild pronation with the elbow flexed. Elbow flexion is not painful but supination is painful. B, To reduce nursemaid's elbow, the forearm is supinated to 90° with the physician's thumb over the radial head to detect the click of reduction. C, If no reduction is felt, the elbow is then hyperflexed until the palpable click reduction is felt over the radial head.

Key references

1. Salter RB, Zaltz C: Anatomic investigation of injury and pathologic anatomy of "pulled elbow" in young children. *Clin Orthop Rel Res* 1971, 77:134–143.

Diagnosis

History

Nonseptic: traumatic (laborers, athletes, paraplegics, elderly persons) is most common; metabolic (gout/pseudogout, rheumatoid arthritis, scleroderma, ankylosing spondylitis, Reiter's syndrome).

Septic: trauma—Direct inoculation of pathogens into superficially situated subcutaneous bursae; olecranon is most commonly involved bursae with septic bursitis (70% of cases).

Physical findings

Nonseptic: usually not painful; fluctuant prominence over elbow; no significant decrease in range of motion; transillumination possible.

Septic: redness, warmth, edema; fluctuance over elbow; drainage may or may not be present; fever; cellulitis; lymphadenopathy.

Imaging and laboratory studies

Radiographs: anteroposterior and lateral of elbow (to rule out foreign body, bony reaction, osteomyelitis).

Laboratory: complete blood count, erythrocyte sedimentation rate. Aspirate (Gram stain, culture and sensitivity, leukocyte cell count with differential, glucose level). Polarized microscopy to identify presence of crystals.

Complications

Missed septic bursitis.

Chronic drainage/wound after bursectomy.

Osteomyelitis if infection is deep.

Decreased range of motion, stiffness.

Differential diagnosis

Nonseptic versus septic.

Rheumatoid nodule.

Gouty tophi.

Tumor (pigmented villonodular synovitis, synovial chondromatosis, synovial sarcoma).

Epidermal inclusion cyst/foreign body reaction.

Septic arthritis (decreased range of motion of the elbow).

Etiology or pathophysiology

Septic versus nonseptic.

Nonseptic.

Trauma is most common cause.

Metabolic factors also responsible.

Occurs in laborers, athletes.

Often secondary to a trivial event.

Epidemiology (risk factors)

Alcoholism.

Steroid use.

Diabetes.

Intravenous drug use.

HIV.

Cancer.

Renal insufficiency.

Dermatitis.

Gout.

Rheumatoid arthritis.

Treatment

Nonsurgical
Nonseptic
Bursal aspiration (diagnostic/therapeutic).
Rest, splinting.
Ice.
Elevation.
Nonsteroidal anti-inflammatory drugs.
Compressive dressings.
Injection of bursae with steroid.
Septic—mild to moderate
Bursal aspiration under aseptic technique.
Oral versus intravenous antibiotics.
Splinting.
Elevation.
Warm compresses.

Surgical
Septic—severe
Incision and drainage.
Intravenous antibiotics.
Bursectomy: for recurrent infections.
Chronically enlarged bursae.

Exercise and activity modification
Keep diabetes well controlled.
Start early intervention if olecranon bursitis is suspected.
Control risk factors.

Treatment aims
Nonseptic
Relieve symptoms.
Prevent septic bursitis.
Prevent recurrence.
Maintain range of motion.
Septic
Control the infection.
Prevent septic arthritis/osteomyelitis.
Maintain range of motion of the elbow.

Prognosis
Nonseptic
Most patients respond to conservative therapy.
Watch for recurrence.
Septic
Prognosis is usually good if condition is treated early.
Patients respond to incision and drainage, oral or intravenous antibiotics, immobilization.

Follow-up and management
Important to follow patients closely for recurrence.
Start range of motion as early as possible (this may be limited by the wound).
Early intervention is the key in both acute and recurrent episodes.

Key references
1. Boutin FJ Sr, Boutin RD, Boutin FJ Jr: Bursitis. In *Operative Orthopaedics* edn 2. Edited by Chapman M. Philadelphia: JB Lippincott; 1993.
2. Ho G Jr, Tile AD, Kaplan SR: Septic bursitis in the prepatellar and olecranon bursae. *Ann Intern Med* 1978, 89:21.
3. McAfee JH, Smith DL: Olecranon and prepatellar bursitis: diagnosis and treatment. *West J Med* 1988, 149:607.
4. Smith DL, McAfee JH, Lucas LM, et al.: Treatment of nonseptic olecranon bursitis: a controlled, blinded prospective trial. *Arch Intern Med* 1989, 149:2527.

Diagnosis

Principles

Plain radiographs are essential to establish or to rule out fractures (Fig. 1).
Radiographs of long bones should include the joint above and below and should
be taken in a standard position—usually an anteroposterior and lateral view will
suffice. Radiographs of children are often confusing because of the growth plates,
especially about the elbow; comparison views with the normal contralateral
extremity are very helpful.

Indications

Obvious deformity of the limb.

Pain about the limb or joint, especially in children.

Inability to use the limb or joint.

Computed Tomography

Principles

Computed tomography provides transverse images of the bone and soft tissues.
Images can also be reconstructed in sagittal and coronal planes for visualization of
complex fracture patterns (Figs. 2 and 3).

Indications

Comminuted fractures about a joint for preoperative planning.

Fractures or suspected fractures of the pelvis.

Fractures or suspected fractures of the cervical, thoracic, or lumbar spine.

Magnetic Resonance Imaging

Principles

Magnetic resonance images best depict soft tissue structures (Fig. 4). Caution
should be exercised in patients with intra-arterial stents, intraocular lenses, and
vascular clips because the magnet causes these devices to be displaced.

Indications

Meniscal tear.

Disk herniation.

Soft tissue tumor.

Intraspinal lesions.

Osteonecrosis of the hip, knee, and shoulder.

Occult fractures of the hip (detection is faster than with bone scanning).

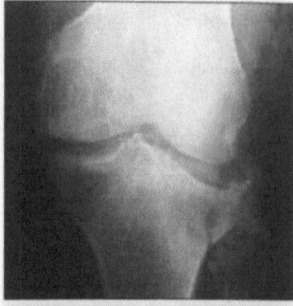

Figure 1. Anteroposterior (AP) plain radiograph of the knee showing a depressed fracture of the lateral tibial plateau.

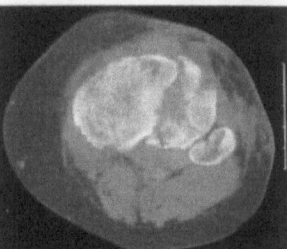

Figure 2. Computed tomography (CT) of case mentioned previously showing comminuted nature of fracture.

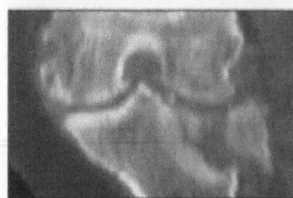

Figure 3. Coronal section reconstruction of the case mentioned previously showing the extent of fracture of the plateau. Coronal and sagittal reconstruction enables the physician to appreciate the three-dimensional nature of complex fractures.

Ultrasonography

Principles
Ultrasonography in orthopedics is primarily used for viewing cystic lesions or vascular structures.

Indications
Ruling out deep venous thrombosis, especially in the vasculature of the thigh.
Evaluating dislocation of the hip in children.

Bone Scanning

Principles
A radioisotope, such as technetium, is injected; active bony lesions take up the isotope; and the lesion is imaged on a full-body scanner (Fig. 5).

Indications
Osteomyelitis.
Multiple bony metastases.
Osteonecrosis (cold lesion).
Stress fractures.

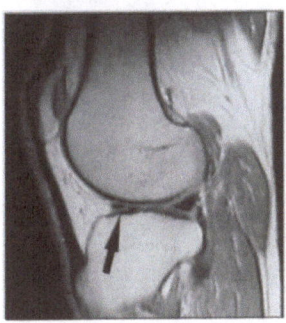

Figure 4. Sagittal magnetic resonance image (MRI) of a different case showing a tear in the anterior horn of the meniscus (*arrow*). MRI best shows soft tissue lesions whereas CT is better at showing bony anatomy.

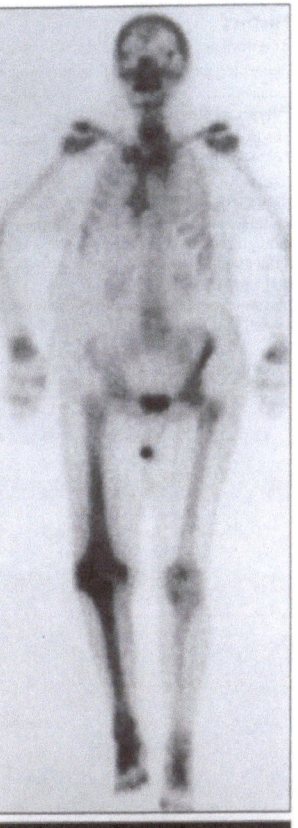

Figure 5. Whole body bone scan showing increased radionucleide uptake in the right tibia in a case of an infected total knee replacement.

Diagnosis

History
Anterior knee pain localized to the tibial tubercle.
Worsening pain with running, jumping, and kneeling.

Physical findings
The tibial tubercle is prominent or is swollen and is markedly tender (Fig. 1).
There should be no knee effusion.

Imaging and laboratory studies
Radiographs: anteroposterior radiographs are unremarkable. Lateral
radiographs show fragmentation and calcification of the tibial tubercle apophysis.
Radiographs are usually used to rule out a more serious abnormality if it is
suspected on initial presentation.

Magnetic resonance imaging: reveals tendonitis and insertion of the tibial tendon,
as well as inflammation of the apophysis.

Complications
With activity, tibial tubercle avulsion may rarely occur.

Differential diagnosis
Patella tendonitis.
Sinding-Larsen-Johansson disease
(apophysitis of the distal pole of
the patella).

Etiology or pathophysiology
This traction apophysitis is thought to
be secondary to repeated microtrauma
and healing.

Epidemiology
Approximately 15% of teenage boys and
10% of teenage girls may be affected.
Bilaterality can occur in up to 55%
of patients.

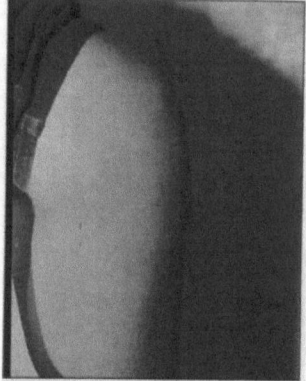

Figure 1. Prominence of tibial tubercle in
patient with Osgood-Schlatter disease.

Treatment

Nonsurgical

Although extended periods away from sports are not recommended, refraining from running and jumping activities for brief periods, usually several days, will control exacerbations of knee pain. Kneeling should be avoided. Brief periods of immobilization may be useful for treating the symptoms of severe acute exacerbations. Nonsteroidal anti-inflammatory drugs are important for controlling pain and inflammation. Local steroid injection is not recommended.

Surgical

After skeletal maturity, a persisting ossicle may occasionally cause continued pain and may have to be removed.

Exercise and activity modification

A marked change of lifestyle and activity for children is not recommended.

Treatment aims
To limit symptoms through resolution of the condition.

Prognosis
The condition is self-limiting, and symptoms resolve at skeletal maturity.

Follow-up and management
Once the natural history of the process has been explained and conservative measures taught to the patient and their family, follow-up is not necessary unless symptoms do not respond to conservative care.

Key references

1. Krause BL, Williams JP, Catterall A: Natural history of Osgood-Schlatter disease. *J Pediatr Orthop* 1990, 10:65–68.
2. Tolo VT: The lower extremity. In *Lovell and Winter's Pediatric Orthopedics*. Edited by Morrissy RT, Weinstein SL. Philadelphia: Lippincott–Raven; 1996:1063–1064.

Diagnosis

Definition
Osteoarthritis is the result of loss of articular cartilage from a joint surface; it primarily affects the major weight-bearing joints of the lower extremities and the spine. As the most common type of arthritis, it is usually progressive and irreversible.

History
Osteoarthritis leads to pain and deformity of the joint and is often associated with stiffness. Pain increases with ambulation and is relieved by rest except in the most advanced cases. Osteophytes may lead to decreased joint motion. The patient may report a history of earlier trauma about the joint (dislocation or fracture) or other surgical procedures that alter the joint mechanics (meniscectomy).

Physical findings
Decreased and painful motion is almost always present, often with painful crepitance as the examiner takes the joint through a range of motion. About the knee, peripheral osteophytes and effusion may be palpable. In osteoarthritis about the knee, the lower extremity is generally in genu varum (bowlegged). When the hip is being examined, the patient should perform a straight-leg raise against resistance. Pain centered within the hip is pathognomonic for abnormality about the hip. Internal and external rotation around the hip are usually limited, and the patient typically walks with the limb externally rotated.

Imaging and laboratory studies
Plain radiographs of the affected joint typically demonstrate loss of cartilage interval, subchondral sclerosis, osteophytes, and the periphery (bone spurs), as well as malalignment of the extremity (Fig. 1).

Complications
Failure to treat osteoarthritis early in its course may lead to severe joint deformity, contracture, and instability.

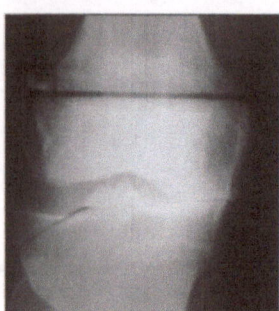

Figure 1. Anteroposterior (AP) plain radiograph of the knee in a patient with severe osteoarthritis of the medial compartment of the knee. Note the nearly complete loss of the cartilage interval in the medial compartment; note the development of subchondral sclerosis, angular deformity, and the medial osteophytes.

Differential diagnosis
Rheumatoid arthritis with secondary degenerative changes (positivity for rheumatoid factor).
Chondrocalcinosis (positivity of joint aspirate for crystals).
Charcot joint (associated with diabetic neuropathy).
Hemophilia.
Hemochromatosis.

Etiology or pathophysiology
Osteoarthritis results from a breakdown of the complicated cartilage matrix, which is composed of cartilage cells, collagen fibrils, proteoglycans, and water (water makes up 60% to 80% of the wet weight). Any factor that disrupts the cartilage surface or places abnormal forces on the cartilage can eventually lead to osteoarthritis, especially in the lower extremity. Factors leading to osteoarthritis about the hip include developmental dysplasia, slipped capital femoral epiphysis, osteonecrosis, and trauma (including fracture and dislocation). Factors leading to osteoarthritis about the knee include fracture, anterior cruciate or medial collateral ligament damage, meniscectomy, and chondrocalcinosis.

Epidemiology
Osteoarthritis is a disease of adults, and its prevalence increases significantly with age. Women are affected more frequently than men. Between 45 and 64 years of age, the prevalence of osteoarthritis in men is 20% compared with 25% in women; between 65 and 74 years of age, the prevalence increases to 38% for men and 52% for women.

Treatment

Nonsurgical

Activity modification: avoid high-impact loading.

Ambulatory aids: cane or crutch.

Bracing: unloader brace for the knee.

Medications: acetaminophen or propoxyphene are the primary recommendations for relieving the pain of osteoarthritis. Nonsteroidal anti-inflammatory drugs may provide relief but cause renal, hepatic, and gastric problems. The use of intra-articular injection of steroids provides only temporary relief. Intra-articular injection of hyaluronic acid is still under investigation but may provide up to 6 months of relief. Glucosamine and chondroitin sulfate have been popularized recently, and both are undergoing larger clinical trials. These drugs have no known side effects.

Exercise: increase muscle tone and range of motion.

Weight loss: reduce force on joints.

Surgical

Arthroscopic debridement—removes loose bodies and trims torn cartilage.

Osteotomy about the knee or hip to redirect forces.

Fusion of affected joints.

Joint replacement of the hip, knee, shoulder, and elbow.

Chondral replacement with cartilage plugs or cultured cartilage cells; still experimental.

Exercise and activity modification

The patient should use a cane on the opposite side of affected hips, same side for affected knees. Crutches should be used if the patient has severe involvement. Water exercises increase motion about the joint and strengthening exercises also should be used. Athletic shoes decrease the impact of hard surfaces and reaching devices lessen bending. See Nonsurgical Treatment section.

Treatment aims

Treatment of osteoarthritis should result in full or near-full return to premorbid function, including the ability to ambulate without pain and perform activities of daily living with minimal restriction.

Prognosis

Treatment of the symptoms of osteoarthritis may provide several months to years of relief. However, once full-thickness cartilage damage is present, the arthritis will continue to progress. Modification of lifestyle, weight loss, and exercise can prolong useful joint function for several years. Corrective osteotomies may provide up to 7 or more years of relief. Total joint replacements routinely function well for 15 years, and some last longer than 20 years. New developments in design may further prolong survival.

Follow-up and management

Patients receiving nonsteroidal anti-inflammatory drugs should be observed carefully for possible renal, gastric, and hepatic side effects. Patients who have undergone total joint replacement should be monitored at least every other year with radiographs to assess the integrity of the replacement.

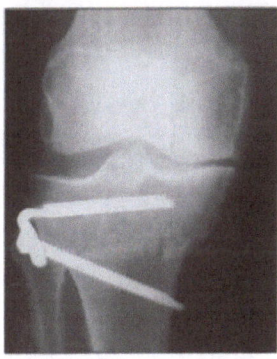

Figure 2. Anteroposterior plain radiograph of the same patient after corrective osteotomy of the tibia and after fixation with an osteotomy plate. Angular deformity has decresed and the medial joint space is wider.

Key references

1. Snider RK: *Essentials of Musculoskeletal Care.* Rosemont, IL: American Academy of Orthopaedic Surgeons; 1997.

2. Simon SR: *Orthopaedic Basic Science.* Rosemont, IL: American Academy of Orthopaedic Surgeons; 1994.

A. Agarwal

Diagnosis

History

Patients with osteoarthritis of the hand generally also manifest arthritis in other areas of the body, such as the hip or knee. Occasionally, the hand may be the only site affected. Patients report stiffness and pain. The pain can be mild to severe and is related to activity. In severe cases, pain can occur at rest. The disorder can manifest itself in one joint, multiple joints of one hand, or both hands. Patients may have deformities in the interphalangeal joints of the hand. The onset is gradual over time and occurs late in life.

Physical findings

Physical examination reveals limitation of motion in the joints of the hand, depending on severity. The joints frequently involved include the distal and proximal interphalangeal joints, and the trapeziometacarpal joint (first or thumb carpometacarpal joint). Most often, patients have nodes (cysts) on their distal interphalangeal joints; these are called Heberden's nodes. They may also have nodes (cysts) on the proximal interphalangeal joints, called Bouchard's nodes. If the thumb carpometacarpal joint is involved, patients may have a painful grind test, subluxation, adduction deformity, weak pinch, and secondary metacarpophalangeal joint hyperextension. All joints of the hand should be evaluated. The metacarpophalangeal joints and the scapho-trapezio-trapezoid joint can also be involved. A secondary tenosynovitis can occur, presenting as carpal tunnel syndrome or flexor tenosynovitis.

Imaging and laboratory studies

Plain radiographs are the only imaging studies necessary. The following laboratory studies can be obtained, primarily to rule out other causes of the pain: complete blood count, erythrocyte sedimentation rate, antinuclear antibody, and rheumatoid factor. If osteomyelitis is in the differential diagnosis, a bone scan or indium scan may have some benefit.

Complications

The major complications from osteoarthritis of the hand are pain and disability.

Differential diagnosis
Rheumatoid arthritis; posttraumatic arthritis; psoriatic arthritis; scleroderma; lupus; crystal arthropathies; gout; pseudogout; osteomyelitis.

Etiology or pathophysiology
Genetics, geography, race, and other environmental factors have been implicated. The pathophysiology is somewhat clearer. Erosion of cartilage, which results in loss of proteoglycans, results in the activation of proteoglycan synthesis. Unfortunately, it also results in an increase in proteases, which can further erode the cartilage. The body attempts to repair itself by chondrocyte proliferation and increased synthesis of chondroitin sulfate. This repair process may produce fibrocartilage that is biomechanically inferior to normal hyaline cartilage. Because many patients have isolated first carpometacarpal joint arthritis, it has been proposed that the cause is mechanical in nature.

Epidemiology
Radiographic studies have shown that almost 90% of adults more than 75 years of age have osteoarthritis. Women are affected more than men. The two most powerful variables in development of osteoarthritis of the hands are age and heredity. The distal interphalangeal joint is involved in 85% of patients, the first carpometacarpal joint in 65%, and the proximal interphalangeal joint in 45%. First carpometacarpal joint arthritis is categorized into four stages according to Eaton's classification. Stage I disease shows only joint space widening due to synovitis or ligament laxity. In stage II disease, the disease progresses to narrowing of the carpometacarpal joint with osteophytes or loose bodies that are less than 2 mm. With marked narrowing of the carpometacarpal joint with subluxation and larger osteophytes, disease has progressed to stage III. Once the scapho-trapezio-trapezoid joint is involved, stage IV disease has been reached. Osteoarthritis can be classified as primary or secondary. Primary osteoarthritis is characterized by Heberden's nodes, Bouchard's nodes, and first carpometacarpal joint involvement. Secondary arthritis is caused by trauma, avascular necrosis, prior inflammatory conditions, and metabolic disorders.

Treatment

Nonsurgical

Nonsteroidal anti-inflammatory drugs are the mainstay for the treatment of osteoarthritis. Hand therapy can be an important part of the treatment plan. Treatment should involve both splinting, activity modification, and patient education and reassurance. Steroid injections may play a role in the treatment.

Surgical

Surgery is indicated only for patients with pain that is unresponsive to nonsurgical treatment or for patients with deformity or instability that impairs function.

Distal interphalangeal joint: if the patient has intractable pain, deformity, or instability with pain, fusion is indicated. It can be performed with Kirschner wires. The index finger should be fused at 10° to 15° and the small finger at 30°. If the cysts or osteophytes are painful or present a cosmetic concern, excision and debridement of the joint can be performed. Arthroplasty is rarely indicated.

Proximal interphalangeal joint: The primary surgical indication is persistent pain; deformity or instability that impairs function is secondary. Stiffness alone is not an indication. If the patient has marked deformity or instability with pain, poor bone stock, or an inadequate flexor or extensor mechanism in the radial digits, fusion is the best option. If persistent pain is present with adequate bone stock, good alignment, and preserved flexor and extensor tendons in the ulnar three fingers, arthroplasty is a good option.

First carpometacarpal joint: The primary surgical indication is persistent pain; deformity or instability that causes disability is a secondary indication. Multiple options are available, and patient factors must be considered. For the high-demand or younger patient with isolated first carpometacarpal joint disease, an arthrodesis should be performed. The overall procedure of choice in many institutions is a total or partial trapezium resection with ligamentous reconstruction and tendon interposition. This procedure can, however, be performed without the ligamentous reconstruction or with silicone interposition. These procedures are usually done for stage III disease. Stabilization of the joint by reconstructing the beak ligament with a strip of flexor carpi radialis tendon is performed in patients with stage I disease if they have the surgical indications noted. Stage II disease is sometimes treated with a metacarpal osteotomy. A panfusion is indicated in stage IV disease.

Exercise and activity modification

Hand therapy is an integral part of nonoperative management.

Treatment aims
To relieve pain and reestablish pain-free motion. The goal of surgical treatment is to relieve pain and ensure a stable digit.

Prognosis
Depends on the joints involved and the severity of the disease.

Follow-up and management
Nonsurgical management is used as needed. Postoperative management requires follow-up, which includes rehabilitation and strengthening. This is especially true for patients who have had arthroplasty.

Key references
1. Pellegrini VD Jr: Osteoarthritis. In *Hand Surgery Update.* Edited by Manske PR. Rosemont, IL: American Academy of Orthopaedic Surgeons. 1994:183–195.

J.D. Mabrey

Diagnosis

Definition
Osteoarthritis of the hip is a direct result of damage to the cartilage surface of the joint.

History
Patients report pain with activity that is relieved by rest. Pain is aggravated by changes in the weather. More severe cases involve catching in the joint and loss of motion.

Physical findings
Patients have decreased range of motion about the hip, especially internal and external rotation. They may walk with a limp, and the affected limb may be shorter than the other limb.

Imaging and laboratory studies
Plain radiographs demonstrate loss of the cartilage interval, osteophytes, and cyst formation. Often there is a large medial osteophyte in the acetabulum.

Complications
Loss of motion.

Pain.

Differential diagnosis
Stress fracture.
Rheumatoid arthritis.

Etiology or pathophysiology
Osteoarthritis of the hip is caused by disruption of the cartilage matrix. It is often secondary to mechanical changes resulting from early hip dysplasia (Fig. 1), slipped capital femoral epiphysis, or trauma.

Epidemiology
Incidence increases with age.

Treatment

Nonsurgical

Cane supported by opposite hand.

Acetaminophen.

Nonsteroidal anti-inflammatory drugs.

Glucosamine/chondroitin sulfate.

Exercise, weight loss, and activity modification.

Surgical

Pelvic or femoral osteotomies in the early stages of the disease to redirect the forces across the hip toward healthier cartilage.

Total hip replacement with a variety of designs, including cemented and porous ingrowth implants.

Exercise and activity modification

Patients should use a cane on the opposite hand of the side to the affected hip. Athletic shoes absorb the impact of walking on hard surfaces. Range-of-motion exercises maintain mobility.

Treatment aims
To maintain pain-free ambulation and activities of daily living.

Prognosis
Limited success with osteotomies. Medications are usually a temporizing measure. Total hip arthroplasties can last 12 to 15 years or longer (Fig. 2).

Follow-up and management
Monitor symptoms as needed. Monitor total hips yearly.

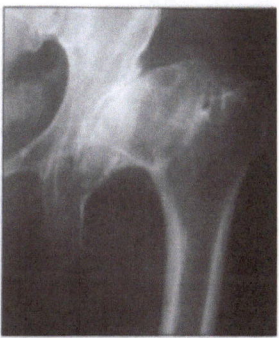

Figure 1. Osteoarthritis of the hip secondary to developmental dysplasia in an adult patient.

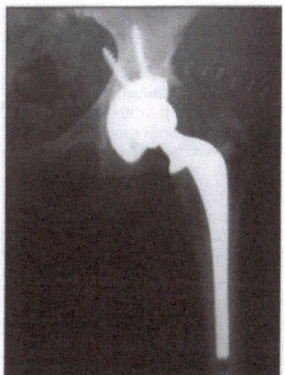

Figure 2. Anteroposterior (AP) radiograph of a total hip arthroplasty. Screws in the acetabulum stabilize the porous-coated cup and help bony ingrowth. The femoral stem is cemented.

Key references
1. Morrey BF: *Joint Replacement Arthroplasty.* Rochester, MN: Mayo Foundation; 1991.

R.M. Campbell, Jr.

Diagnosis

History
Patients with hematogenous osteomyelitis present with severe pain of the affected bone, often with constitutional symptoms of malaise, fever, chills, and loss of appetite. The child may limp, refuse to walk, or cease using the affected part.

Physical findings
The limp is antalgic with shortened stance phase. The infected bone is tender, and the adjacent joint may have a sympathetic effusion. There may be fullness or frank swelling of the extremity. Erythema is rare.

Imaging and laboratory studies
An anteroposterior and lateral radiograph of the long bone is taken. Osteomyelitis that has been symptomatic for less than 10 days only deep soft tissue edema; later areas of lucency develop in the bone with periosteal calcification. Most hematogenous osteomyelitis is seen in the metaphysis; the exception is diaphyseal osteomyelitis caused by salmonella, which sometimes occurs in patients with sickle cell disease. Early in the disease, when radiographs are negative, technetium bone scans may show increased uptake of isotope in areas of active infection. Computed tomography scans may show increased marrow density in early cases and confirm periosteal calcification in later cases (Fig. 1). Magnetic resonance imaging scans are useful in equivocal cases because they show early marrow changes and any subperiosteal abscess.

Laboratory studies should include complete blood count with erythrocyte sedimentation rate, blood cultures, measurement of C-reactive protein levels, and urinalysis. An increased leukocyte count, a shift to the left in the differential, elevated sedimentation rate, and elevated C-reactive protein level support the diagnosis. The involved bone should be aspirated for Gram stain and culture.

Complications
Pathologic fractures through areas of weakened bone can occur in untreated osteomyelitis (Fig. 2). Septic arthritis of the adjacent joint can develop if a metaphyseal bone abscess ruptures into a joint space. Growth can be disturbed or arrested with severe metaphyseal infection.

Differential diagnosis
Occult fracture; bone infarct in sickle cell anemia; tumor; fibrous dysplasia; scurvy; leukemia; neoplasm.

Etiology
In hematogenous osteomyelitis of childhood, transient bacteremia may seed the metaphyseal regions of the long bones, where circulation is sluggish in the venous sinusoids adjacent to the growth plate. Microabscesses form and destroy bone, and pus spreads through the fenestrated cortex of the metaphysis to collect under the periosteum. Osteomyelitis due to penetrating trauma or open fracture does occur in children but is rare. Incidental trauma is noted in a significant percentage of cases of hematologous osteomyelitis in children, but it is unclear whether there is a causal relationship. The most common causative organisms depend on the age of the patient:
Neonates: *Staphylococcus aureus*, group B streptococci, enteric bacilli.
1 month to 3 years: *S. aureus*, streptococci, *Haemophilus influenzae*.
Older than 3 years: *S. aureus*, streptococci, *Pseudomonas* species.

Epidemiology
Osteomyelitis has a peak incidence in the last part of the first decade of life and is more common in boys. There are seasonal differences, with more cases reported in late summer and early autumn.

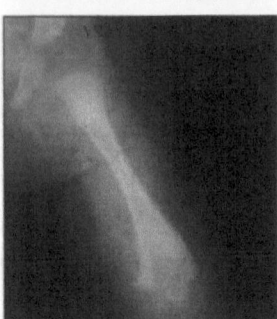

Figure 1. A patient with late diagnosis of osteomyelitis. Radiographs show interosseous abscess of the distal femur with bone destruction and periosteal calcification.

Treatment

Nonsurgical

If aspirates are negative for gross purulence, the patient receives intravenous therapy with a broad-spectrum antibiotic and is monitored for clinical response. In patients older than 1 year, *S. aureus* is probably the causative organism, and intravenous oxacillin (150 mg/kg/d, administered every 6 hours) or intravenous methicillin (150 mg/kg/d, administered every 6 hours) is a good choice for initial coverage. A cephalosporin is also a good choice, especially if the patient is allergic to penicillin, and both intravenous cefazolin (100 mg/kg/d, administered every 8 hours) and intravenous cefuroxime (100 to 150 mg/kg/d, administered every 8 hours) can be used. If later cultures are positive, the antibiotic is changed to one that is specific for that organism. However, 30% to 50% of cases of osteomyelitis are culture-negative, and those patients must continue to receive broad-spectrum antibiotics. While they are receiving intravenous antibiotics, patients are monitored for decreased tenderness and swelling of the extremity, defervescence, return of appetite, and ability to use the extremity normally. With successful treatment, levels of C-reactive protein decrease within days, but sedimentation rates tend to stay elevated for weeks. Once improvement is seen clinically, discharge to outpatient status is considered.

Conversion to oral antibiotics is possible if the following criteria are satisfied: the organism is isolated and an oral antibiotic is available for its treatment, bactericidal levels of oral antibiotics to the isolated organism are obtainable, the patient can tolerate the antibiotic, and there is reasonable assurance that the family will comply to complete a course of treatment. The choice of oral antibiotic depends on culture results. Antibiotic treatment can last from 3 weeks for mild cases to 6 weeks for more severe disease. Serial determinations of C-reactive protein levels and sedimentation rate assist in decisions about length of treatment.

Surgical

If gross purulence is seen on the bone aspirates obtained at presentation or if clinical improvement does not occur within 48 hours after the start of treatment for aspiration-negative patients, incision and drainage of the bone are indicated in addition to antibiotic treatment.

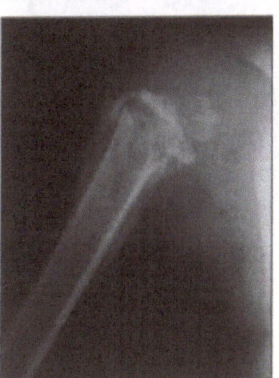

Figure 2. A young patient with septic arthritis of the shoulder underwent treatment with serial needle aspirations but treatment was complicated by a pathologic fracture of the proximal humerus. The fracture resulted from associated osteomyelitis of the proximal humerus.

Key references

1. Morrissy RT: Bone and joint sepsis in children. *Instructional Course Lectures.* Rosemont, IL: American Academy of Orthopaedic Surgeons; 1982:49.

OSTEONECROSIS   J.D. Mabrey

Diagnosis

Definition
Osteonecrosis (also known as *avascular necrosis*) most commonly affects the hip but may also affect the proximal humerus, knee, and talus.

History
Nonspecific symptoms.

Pain, limp, decreased range of motion.

No symptoms in early stages.

Risk factors include the following:

Trauma (dislocation).

Sickle-cell disease.

Corticosteroids given for transplants.

Alcohol abuse.

Decompression sickness.

Physical findings
Affects both hips in 50% of cases.

Pain on motion.

Imaging and laboratory studies
Radiographs: in early stages may be normal; in later stages, shows mottling composed of areas of sclerosis and radiolucency and collapse of femoral head,

Magnetic resonance imaging (MRI): the best single method for early diagnosis of osteonecrosis; shows decreased signal intensity in the femoral head (Fig. 1).

Bone scanning: no longer recommended except when patients cannot undergo MRI.

Complications
Collapse of the femoral head if treatment is not initiated soon enough.

Progression of contralateral lesion if all attention is focused on symptomatic hip.

Differential diagnosis

Sickle cell crisis in patients at risk.

Osteoarthritis.

Spinal abnormality.

Bursitis.

Bone marrow edema, a precursor to osteonecrosis that may resolve spontaneously within 6 months.

Etiology or pathophysiology

Traumatic disruption of blood supply.

Intravascular coagulation.

Intraosseous hypertension.

Fat embolism.

Hemoglobinopathies.

Epidemiology

Underlying diagnosis in 5% to 18% of the 500,000 total hips performed yearly, worldwide.

10,000 to 20,000 new cases each year in United States.

Secondary to dislocation in 26% of cases.

Incidence in renal transplant recipients, 5%.

Incidence in heart transplant recipients, 3%.

Incidence is 10% to 17% in patients with sickle cell anemia.

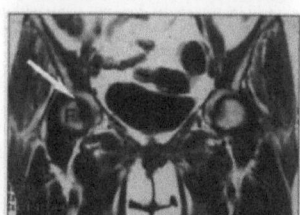

Figure 1. Coronal section of magnetic resonance imaging (MRI) of a patient with steroid-induced osteonecrosis of the femoral head (F). Note the loss of signal (dark area—*arrow*) within the superior region of the head.

Treatment

Nonsurgical
Limited weight-bearing has no place in the treatment of osteonecrosis of the femoral head.

External electrical stimulation may be of some use.

Avoidance of corticosteroids or alcohol.

Surgical
Core decompression.

Osteotomy.

Vascularized fibular graft.

Total hip replacement after collapse.

Treatment aims
Preservation of the femoral head.

Prognosis
Core decompression arrests the process in approximately 75% of cases. Vascularized fibular grafting may be successful in severe cases. Total hip arthroplasty eliminates the pain.

Follow-up and management
Asymptomatic osteonecrosis should be followed carefully and core decompression offered when symptoms appear.
Knee: radionuclide bone scan shows focally increased uptake before the radiographs are abnormal. Many patients have a benign course followed by resolution of symptoms. Conservative management is indicated initially.
Shoulder: few patients with sickle cell anemia require any treatment. More than half of steroid-induced cases of osteonecrosis require shoulder replacement.
Talus: the incidence of osteonecrosis is greatest in fractures with the most displacement. The Hawkins sign (patchy subchondral osteoporosis seen 6 to 8 weeks after injury) signifies revascularization and a good prognosis.

Key references
1. Ecker ML, Lotke PA: Spontaneous osteonecrosis of the knee. J Am Acad Orthop Surg 1994, 2:173–178.
2. Hattrup SJ: Indications, technique, and results of shoulder arthroplasty in osteonecrosis. Orthop Clin North Am 1998, 29:445–451.
3. Mont MA, Carbone JJ, Fairbank AC: Core decompression versus nonoperative management for osteonecrosis of the hip. Clin Orthop 1996, 324:169–178.
4. Urbaniak JR, Jones JF: Osteonecrosis: Etiology, Diagnosis, and Treatment. Rosemont, IL: American Academy of Orthopaedic Surgeons; 1997.

Diagnosis

History

Osteoporosis is often called the "silent disease" because bone loss occurs without symptoms. People may not know that they have osteoporosis until their bones become so weak that a sudden strain, bump, or fall causes a hip fracture or a vertebra to collapse. Risk factors for osteoporosis include the following: anorexia, diet low in calcium and vitamin D, use of glucocorticoids or phenytoin, inactive lifestyle or extended bed rest, cigarette smoking, excessive use of alcohol, northern European descent, early menopause.

Physical findings

Collapsed vertebra may initially be felt or seen in the form of severe back pain, loss of height, or spinal deformities such as kyphosis or severely stooped posture.

Imaging and laboratory studies

Imaging

Radiographs: detect bone loss only after approximately 30% to 50% of the bone mineral is lost. Anteroposterior and lateral radiographs of the thoracic and lumbar spines are useful in detecting fractures of the vertebrae (Fig. 1).

Bone densitometry: single- and dual-energy x-ray absorptiometry are the most widely used methods of bone densitometry. Radiation dose is minimal (1 to 3 mrem). Repeated studies must be done on the same machine each time to be meaningful (Fig. 2).

Bone biopsy: transilial bone biopsy can be done on an outpatient basis. Oral tetracycline must be given before biopsy to label bone.

Laboratory

Complete blood count.

Measurement of electrolytes, blood urea nitrogen, creatinine, calcium, phosphorus, protein, albumin, and liver enzymes.

Protein electrophoresis.

Thyroid function tests.

Testosterone (men only).

24-hour urine for calcium and pyridinium cross-links.

Serum: 25-hydroxyvitamin D_3, 1,25-dihydroxyvitamin D_3, parathyroid hormone, osteocalcin.

Urine: immunoelectrophoresis, Bence Jones protein.

Complications

Fracture.

Pain.

Deformity of spine.

Differential diagnosis

Osteomalacia.

Endocrine disorders: Cushing's disease, diabetes, hyperparathyroidism, iatrogenic (caused by glucocorticoid treatment).

Disuse disorders: immobilization, paralysis.

Neoplastic: multiple myeloma, leukemia.

Nutritional: anorexia, high-phosphate diet, low-calcium diet, alcoholism.

Hematologic: sickle cell anemia, thalassemia.

Collagen disorders: homocystinuria, osteogenesis imperfecta.

Hyperthyroidism.

Epidemiology

Bone mass reaches its peak between the ages of 16 and 25. The more bone present, the less chance of developing osteoporosis. Men lose bone at a rate of approximately 0.3% per year; the rate in women is 0.5% per year, accelerating to 2% to 3% per year after menopause. This accelerated rate lasts for 6 to 10 years.

Treatment

Nonsurgical

Calcium: age 11 to 24 years, 1200 to 1500 mg/d; 25 to 64 years, 1000 mg/d; women not receiving estrogen replacement therapy age 51 or older, 1500 mg/d; 65 years or older, 1500 mg/d.

Vitamin D: 400 to 800 IU/d in conjunction with calcium.

Estrogen replacement therapy: has been shown to reduce bone loss, increase bone density in both the spine and hip, and reduce the risk for hip and spinal fractures in postmenopausal women.

Alendronate: one of the bisphosphonates compounds that inhibit bone breakdown and slow bone removal; it has been shown to increase bone density and decrease the risk for fractures at both the hip and spine. Must be taken on an empty stomach.

Raloxifene: one of a new class of drugs called selective estrogen receptor modulators (SERMs) that appear to prevent bone loss at the spine, hip, and total body. Raloxifene's effect on the spine does not seem to be as powerful as the effect of estrogen replacement therapy or alendronate, but its effects on the hip and total body are similar. Like estrogens, SERMs produce changes in blood lipids that may protect against heart disease, although the effects are not as potent as that of estrogen. Unlike estrogens, SERMs do not appear to stimulate uterine or breast tissue.

Calcitonin: available as an injection or nasal spray. In women who are at least 5 years beyond menopause, calcitonin slows bone loss, increases spinal bone density, and, according to anecdotal reports, relieves the pain associated with bone fractures.

Surgical

No specific treatment. Physicians may recommend bone biopsy for diagnosis. Surgery may be used to treat resultant fractures.

Exercise and activity modification

Exercise: gentle exercises with avoidance of sudden strains prevent further bone mineral loss.

Diet: calcium and vitamin D as noted above.

Treatment aims
To maintain or increase bone mass, prevent bone loss, and prevent fracture.

Prognosis
Osteoporosis is best treated by preventing bone loss. Once the symptoms of osteoporosis have appeared, it is almost impossible to return to a normal bone mass.

Follow-up and management
Monitor bone mass every 2 years in postmenopausal women to assess the effects of treatment or to screen for osteoporosis.

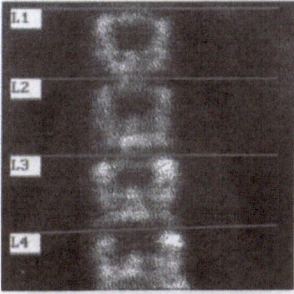

Figure 2. Dual energy x-ray absoptiometry of the lumbar spine.

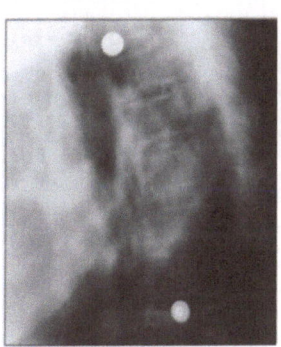

Figure 1. Lateral radiograph of the thoracic spine in a patient with severe osteoporosis resulting from steroid use. Note the multiple wedge compression fractures of the vertebrae.

Key references
1. Simon SR: *Orthopaedic Basic Science.* Rosemont, IL: American Academy of Orthopaedic Surgeons; 1994.
2. Kasser JR: *Orthopaedic Knowledge Update 5.* Rosemont, IL: American Academy of Orthopaedic Surgeons; 1996.

Diagnosis

History
Patients report recent traumatic injury to the hand. They may have sustained the fracture in an occupational injury or sports. A crush injury to the hand can also result in a phalangeal fracture. Often these injuries have open wounds.

Physical findings
Patients with a fracture of the phalanx will have swelling, loss of motion, and tenderness to palpation in the injured finger. The findings vary with the level involved. With distal phalanx fractures, an associated nail and nailbed injury may also be present. Some may have an obvious rotational or angular deformity. An assessment of this angular or rotational deformity is crucial for determining the appropriate treatment. Because of the mechanism of injury in these cases, 30% to 50% are open fractures.

Imaging and laboratory studies
Three radiographic views—anteroposterior, lateral, and oblique—of the affected digit should be taken. Hand radiographs are not needed unless other fingers are also involved (Fig. 1). Individual radiographs of the digit provide better detail and enlargement of the injury (Fig. 2).

Complications
Malunion is probably the most common complication with nonoperative treatment. Infection can be a concern in open injuries. In addition, depending on the level of phalanx involved, stiffness of the adjacent joint can be a problem after immobilization. If the joint is involved in the fracture, posttraumatic arthritis may be a problem.

Differential diagnosis
Fractures of the phalanx are usually very straightforward when it comes to diagnosis. However, the digit can swell in non-traumatic conditions, such as tenosynovitis or a pulp infection in the finger. Severe rheumatoid arthritis or osteoarthritis may also present with deformity and swelling. Other traumatic conditions include mallet finger and dislocations of the interphalangeal joints.

Etiology or pathophysiology
Phalangeal fractures can occur anywhere along the length of the phalanx. The usual mechanism is a direct crush to the involved finger. A twisting injury also accounts for a large portion of these fractures. Axial loading injuries to the digits can result in phalangeal fractures. Distal phalanx fractures are caused by a crush mechanism in most cases and therefore have an associated nailbed injury.

Epidemiology
Hand fractures account for approximately 10% of all adult fractures. Of these, 70% involve the phalanges. The other 30% are metacarpal fractures. More than 50% of hand fractures are work related. The border digits are the most commonly involved, and the distal phalanx is the phalanx most commonly injured, with an incidence approaching 65%. The proximal phalanx is injured in 20% of cases, followed in frequency by the middle phalanx (15% of cases).
Fractures can be intra-articular, extra-articular, or fracture-dislocations of the joint. The intra-articular fractures are condylar fractures, single, bicondylar, or osteochondral. Fracture-dislocations can be volar or dorsal. Extra-articular fractures occur at the neck, shaft, or base. The fractures at the base tend to angulate with the apex dorsal, while those at the neck tend to have apex volar angulation.

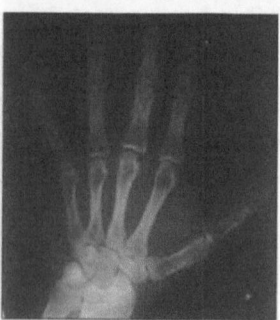

Figure 1. Anteroposterior (AP) view of a fracture of the proximal phalanx of the long finger. The detail is somewhat obscure.

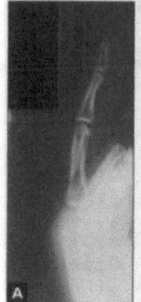 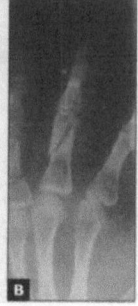 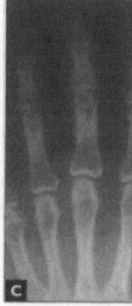

Figure 2. A, The lateral, **B,** oblique, and **C,** anteroposterior views of the digit enlarge the image and provide better fracture detail. The figures show the long finger proximal phalanx with an oblique fracture of the shaft.

Treatment

Nonsurgical

If the injury can be reduced in a closed manner, then splinting or buddy taping will suffice as the treatment. If any of the conditions mentioned under Surgical Treatment are met, operative treatment is indicated. Almost all distal phalanx fractures that are extra-articular can be treated with splinting, with or without closed reduction. If a subungual hematoma is present with an intact nail, pain can be relieved by decompressing the nail with either a heated needle or battery-operated electrocautery unit. Some authors have advocated removal of the nail and repair of the nailbed. This treatment is somewhat debatable.

Surgical

The decision to operate is based on many variables: deformity, stability, amount of joint involvement, associated soft tissue injury, and displacement. For fractures and fracture-dislocations with significant joint involvement greater than 30% or greater than 1 mm of displacement, open reduction and internal fixation or closed reduction and percutaneous pinning are the best options. If reduction in extra-articular fractures cannot be obtained or maintained, open or closed reduction with stabilization is required.

In general, if any of the following conditions are met, surgical intervention is indicated: failure of closed reduction to maintain length, rotation, and angulation; loss of joint congruity in intra-articular fractures; unstable fractures with associated soft tissue injuries; multiple fractures.

Surgical options include closed reduction and percutaneous pinning with Kirschner wires. Open reduction and internal fixation may be needed if closed reduction fails. This can be AO/ASIF minifragment screws or plates, wire techniques, or Kirschner wires. The proximal and middle phalanx should be approached through a midline dorsal (Fig. 3) or midaxial incision. External fixation of these injuries can be used in open injuries with gross contamination. Special fixators are available or Kirschner wires can be used as an external fixator apparatus.

Exercise and activity modification

Activities are usually restricted to patient tolerance and occupation because of the need for splinting of the hand.

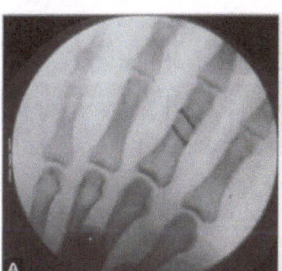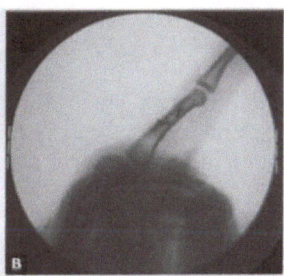

Figure 3. Open reduction and internal fixation were performed through a dorsal midline incision. Two minifragment lag screws were used to fix the fracture. A, Anteroposterior (AP) and B, lateral views are shown.

Treatment aims
To restore full use of the hand without pain or stiffness.

Prognosis
Most phalanx fractures heal uneventfully with excellent return of function. Open injuries tend to have stiffness problems. The severity of the associated soft tissue injury is usually the limiting factor in terms of prognosis.

Follow-up and management
If closed treatment is instituted, splinting can be used for 4 weeks. After this period, buddy taping with active motion can usually be started. Some injuries that are extremely stable may be buddy taped with immediate active motion. Postoperative management is similar, with immediate splinting after surgery. Depending on the fixation used, early range of motion can be started. If plates and screws were used and stable fixation achieved, immediate active motion can begin. Kirschner wires may limit some active motion. These pins can usually be pulled after 4 weeks, followed by motion.

Key references
1. Hastings H: Unstable metacarpal and phalangeal fracture treatment with screws and plates. *Clin Orthop* 1987, 214:37–52.
2. Maitra A, Burdett-Smith P: The conservative management of proximal phalangeal fractures of the hand. *J Hand Surg* 1991, 16B:137–140.

Diagnosis

History

Plantar fasciitis is often insidious in onset but can be associated with a recent history of increased physical activity. Patients primarily report pain on the plantar medial aspect of the heel. The pain is particularly severe with the first few steps in the morning after getting out of bed or after arising from a seated position. The pain subsides with continued walking but worsens with excessive standing and walking during the day. The pain can be relieved by getting off one's feet and taking nonsteroidal anti-inflammatory drugs. The condition is rarely associated with numbness or tingling on the sole of the foot.

Physical findings

The plantar medial aspect of the calcaneus at the origin of the plantar fascia is almost always tender, often severely, to palpation. Mild swelling sometimes occurs in this area, and sensation to light touch over the heel pad may, albeit rarely, be slightly decreased.

Imaging and laboratory studies

A lateral radiograph of the heel sometimes demonstrates a "heel spur" (Fig. 1). This calcification or ossification of the origin of the plantar fascia indicates chronic inflammation of the plantar fascia but is not responsible for the pain. Indeed, 20% to 30% of the normal adult population will have a "heel spur" on routine radiographs. In chronic cases, a technetium-99 bone scan shows increased localized uptake at the site of origin of the plantar fascia.

Complications

Chronic inflammation of the plantar fascia sometimes leads to rupture of the fascia, producing a chronic flatfoot deformity.

Differential diagnosis

Several conditions may mimic plantar fasciitis: Achilles tendonitis, retrocalcaneal bursitis, stress fracture of the calcaneus, arthritis of the subtalar joint, and seronegative spondyloarthropathies, such as ankylosing spondylitis or Reiter's syndrome.

Etiology or pathophysiology

Chronic inflammation of the plantar fascia where it originates from the tuberosity of the calcaneus results in small tears and degeneration of the fascia. Even limited weight-bearing activities aggravate the inflammation and cause the symptoms to persist.

Epidemiology

Plantar fasciitis usually affects middle-aged adults. It is somewhat more common in overweight, middle-aged persons but it occurs in athletes who participate in repetitive, stressful activities.

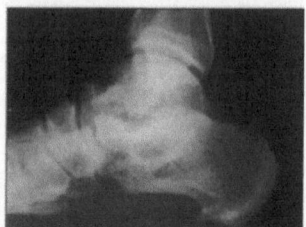

Figure 1. Lateral radiograph showing a heel spur caused by ossification of the origin of the plantar fascia.

Treatment

Nonsurgical

Many different methods have been used to control the symptoms related to plantar fasciitis, which is a self-limited disease—one that almost always resolves with time. Therefore, nonoperative treatment should be given to control symptoms until the disease runs its course. The first line of defense consists of the use of cushioned heel cups, heel-cord stretching exercises, and the use of a night splint designed to hold the foot and ankle at a right angle during sleep. The night splint prevents overnight contracture of the heel cord and plantar fascia and often is very effective at relieving morning pain. Nonsteroidal anti-inflammatory drugs often alleviate the patient's symptoms. The next phase of treatment for recalcitrant plantar fasciitis is a local injection of xylocaine and dexamethasone suspension, such as Celestone Soluspan (Schering, Kenilworth, NJ). Recalcitrant symptoms often respond to complete rest in the form of immobilization achieved through a short-leg walking cast for 6 to 8 weeks.

Surgical

Surgical treatment is reserved for the very small percentage of patients who do not respond to prolonged (longer than 6 months) nonsurgical treatment. A subtotal plantar fascial release combined with decompression of the first branch of the lateral plantar nerve is the current preferred surgical treatment. Complete release of the plantar fascia should be avoided because doing so significantly alters the mechanics of gait and will create a flatfoot deformity.

Exercise and activity modification

Young athletic patients may need to avoid high-impact activities, such as jogging, that seem to aggravate the symptoms. For patients who stand and walk on a concrete surface, the use of a carpet or rubber matting may help relieve chronic heel soreness.

Treatment aims
To control the patient's symptoms during the 6- to 9-month duration of this self-limited disease. In almost all cases, this goal can be accomplished through nonsurgical means.

Prognosis
Generally the prognosis for full recovery is very good. Chronic inflammation of the plantar fascia sometimes results in rupture. Although rupture may relieve the patient's symptoms, it also flattens the longitudinal arch of the foot, which may cause other foot problems in the future.

Follow-up and management
Once plantar fasciitis occurs in one foot, it is not uncommon for symptoms to later develop on the opposite side. Activity and shoewear modification may be very effective at preventing such an occurrence.

Key references
1. Gill H: Plantar fasciitis: diagnosis and conservative management. *J Am Acad Orthop Surg* 1997, 5:109–117.

Diagnosis

History

In elderly persons, fractures result from mild to moderate trauma.

In younger persons, fractures are caused by high-energy trauma.

Fractures may occur from a direct blow to side of shoulder.

Electric shock or convulsive episode may cause a fracture-dislocation (posterior).

Patients report pain after acute trauma.

Physical findings

Pain, swelling, tenderness about the shoulder.

Increased pain around greater tuberosity.

Crepitus may occur with motion.

Ecchymosis (24 to 48 hours after injury).

Detailed neurovascular examination is paramount (the nerve most commonly injured is the axillary nerve).

More than 50% of fracture-dislocations are missed on initial examination (these can be identified by loss of contour of shoulder).

Imaging and laboratory studies

Trauma series: anteroposterior, scapular Y view, and axillary lateral view.

Axillary view is critical for tuberosity displacement and allows assessment of glenoid articular surface and the glenohumeral relationship.

Neer classification: based on four fragments of and their relationship to one another—humeral head; greater tuberosity; lesser tuberosity; humeral shaft.

When any fragment is displaced more than 1 cm or is angulated more than 45°, it is considered displaced.

If unable to obtain adequate radiographs, computed tomography can be helpful in the assessment of proximal humerus fractures.

Complications

Acute vascular injury: axillary artery.

If vascular injury is suspected, angiography should be done.

Brachial plexus injury (6% of cases).

Axillary nerve is most commonly affected.

Chest injury: pneumothorax and hemothorax.

Late frozen shoulder.

Avascular necrosis: stiff, painful joint; 3% to 14% incidence with 3-part fracture; 15% to 34% incidence with 4-part fracture.

Malunion and glenohumeral arthritis.

Nonunion.

Differential diagnosis

If radiograph shows no fracture:

Hemorrhagic bursitis.

Traumatic rotator cuff tear.

Dislocation.

Acromioclavicular separation.

Calcific tendinitis.

Etiology or pathophysiology

Traumatic: fall on outstretched arm or direct impact to shoulder.

Epidemiology

4% to 5% of all fractures.

More common in elderly persons.

45% of humeral fractures.

Male-to-female ratio, 2:1.

More common in patients with significant osteoporosis.

Treatment

Nonsurgical

Treatment for nondisplaced or minimally displaced 2-part fractures.

Sling.

Pendulum exercises when tolerated.

Strengthening can begin when radiograph shows healing.

Surgical

Percutaneous pinning: after closed reduction, percutaneous pinning is useful for unstable 2-part surgical neck fractures.

Open reduction and internal fixation: displaced 2- and 3-part fractures.

4-part fracture (ORIF for this type generally yields poor results, but it may be indicated in younger patients).

Prosthetic replacement for some 3-part proximal humerus fractures, especially elderly patients with osteoporotic bone and all 4-part fractures.

Exercise and activity modification

As described in nonsurgical treatment.

Treatment aims
Fracture healing.
Range of motion.

Prognosis
Low nonunion rate.
Beware of associated injuries.

Follow-up and rehabilitation
When fracture and fracture repair is stable, early rehabilitation can be initiated.
3-phase system of rehabilitation devised by Hughes and Neer:
First phase (up to 6 weeks):
Passive-assistive exercises.
2nd phase (6 weeks):
Active and early resistance.
3rd phase (3 months):
Maintenance program.
Advanced stretching and strengthening.

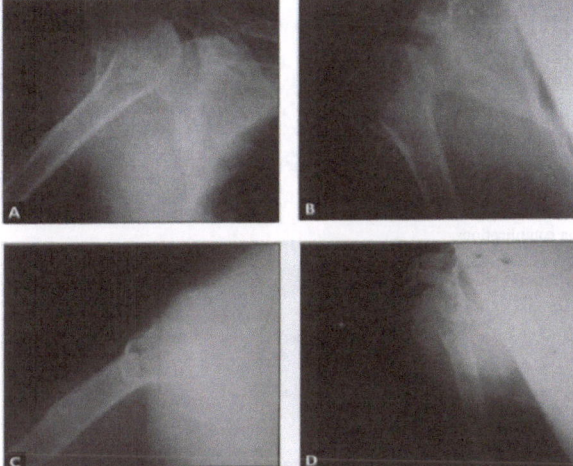

Figure 1. Radiographs of proximal humerus fracture. A and B, Anteroposterior (AP) views, C, Axillary lateral view, D, Scapula Y view.

Diagnosis

History

Most patients who sustain radial head fractures present with a history of falling. Others may have suffered a direct blow to the elbow, such as in an altercation. The injury may be associated with an elbow dislocation or wrist injury.

Physical findings

Patients usually have pain with motion, which is limited. There is associated swelling depending on the severity of the injury. Physical examination of the soft tissue around the elbow and examination of the wrist are key components of the overall evaluation. Valgus instability of the elbow may be present because of associated rupture of the medial collateral ligament. Palpation of the forearm and resultant tenderness may indicate injury to the interosseous membrane. Wrist pain also may indicate distal radioulnar joint (DRUJ) instability. Injury to the interosseous membrane and triangular fibrocartilage at the DRUJ with a radial head fracture result in axial instability of the forearm and subluxation of the DRUJ. This lesion is known as the Essex-Lopresti injury.

Imaging and laboratory studies

Plain radiographs of the elbow (anteroposterior and lateral views) are diagnostic of the injury (Fig. 1). A third view, the radiocapitellar view, can be helpful as well. Wrist and forearm radiographs should be taken to rule any associated abnormality. Computed tomography can be helpful for preoperative planning for comminuted fractures.

Complications

The biggest complication can result from the failure to diagnose an associated Essex-Lopresti lesion or medial collateral ligament rupture. In these injuries, preservation of the radiocapitellar articulation is crucial. If these injuries are not recognized and treated by excision of the radial head, proximal migration of the radius (with Essex-Lopresti lesion) or valgus instability of the elbow (with medial collateral ligament rupture) would ensue. Failure of the hardware, heterotopic ossification, and posttraumatic arthritis are other complications.

Differential diagnosis

Other fractures around the elbow can mimic radial head fractures. A septic joint or neuropathic joint can present with acute swelling as well, but the associated traumatic event may be absent.

Etiology or pathophysiology

Most injuries are the result of a fall on the pronated outstretched arm. A mechanical force is directed throughout the wrist and along the interosseous membrane to the radiocapitellar joint. An associated valgus force is also usually present. As a result, the energy is concentrated on this half of the joint and a radial head fracture occurs. A direct blow to the elbow with an associated valgus force can also occur, and an elbow dislocation may be present.

Epidemiology

Radial head fractures account for 20% of all elbow fractures. Mason classified these injuries into three types. A Type I fracture is nondisplaced. Type II injuries are marginal fractures with displacement. A Type III fracture is comminuted and involves the whole head. An additional category, Type IV, was added later; this fracture is accompanied by an elbow dislocation.

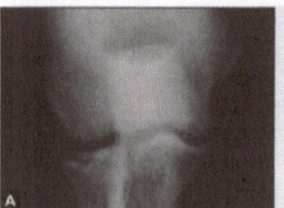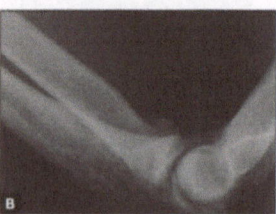

Figure 1. A, Anteroposterior (AP) and B, lateral view of a Mason Type II radial head fracture.

Treatment

Nonsurgical

Early emergency department treatment of these injuries is greatly facilitated by aspiration of the joint and instillation of an anesthetic (lidocaine without epinephrine, with or without Marcaine) into the joint. This both relieves pain and allows examination for a block to motion. All Type I fractures should be treated with initial splinting, followed by early active range of motion. Type II fractures that have no mechanical block to motion can be treated in a similar fashion or can be treated surgically. The decision to operate on a Type II fracture should be based on the patient's expectations and condition.

Surgical

Most Type II and all Type III fractures are best treated by surgical intervention. Type II fractures can be treated with open reduction and internal fixation (ORIF), if the fragment is large enough, or by excision. Excision can be of a small piece or of the entire head if the fracture pattern is not amenable to fixation. Delayed excision of the radial head can also be performed if nonoperative treatment fails. An ORIF procedure can be performed via a Kocher incision using Herbert screws, biodegradable screws, or countersunk AO/ASIF screws (Fig. 2). Plate fixation may be needed from the AO/ASIF hand or mini-fragment sets. Type III fractures are best managed by early radial head excision. To decrease the incidence of heterotopic ossification, excision should be performed within 24 to 48 hours. If there is associated valgus instability of the elbow or an Essex-Lopresti lesion, preservation of the radial head is crucial. If the injury is not amenable to saving the radial head, prosthetic replacement of the radial head should be performed along with associated ligament repair. The prosthesis can consist of be silicone or vitallium. Each material has its associated problems. The silicone prosthesis can be removed 6 to 12 months later. The metal prosthesis can be left in but should be removed at the first sign of loosening, fragmentation, capitellar wear, or dislocation.

Exercise and activity modification

Limit the patient's activities for at least 6 weeks. During this time use aggressive therapy to restore elbow motion. Heavy lifting is usually restricted.

Treatment aims

To restore pain-free motion to the elbow joint without compromising the stability of the joint itself. Complications of arthritis and heterotopic ossification should be avoided.

Prognosis

The prognosis for Type I injuries is generally excellent by 2 to 3 months. These patients regain all their motion and have little to no residual disability. The Type II injuries treated with ORIF usually have good to excellent results, although they lose some terminal extension and some rotation. The Type III injuries treated with excision only lose about 15° of rotation or less. They do, however, lose some pronation and supination strength. In 70% to 80% of cases in which delayed excision is indicated, pain is relieved and function improves.

Follow-up and management

All injuries need a short duration of immobilization with a posterior splint. Early active and active-assist motion is started after both nonsurgical and surgical treatment. This is usually started in the initial 7 to 10 days after injury. A sling can be used for comfort. Indomethacin, either 25 mg orally three times daily or 75 mg of the slow-release formulation every day, can be given to help minimize the incidence of heterotopic ossification.

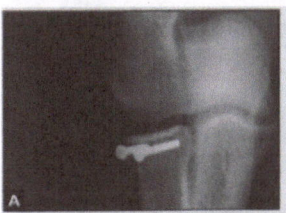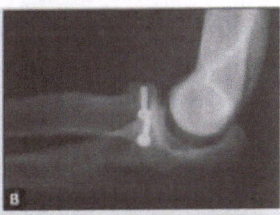

Figure 2. A, Anteroposterior (AP) and B, lateral view of the fracture after open reduction and internal fixation using two minifragment screws. The joint surface has been anatomically restored and the step-off eliminated.

Key references

1. Davidson PA, Moseley JB Jr, Tullos HS: Radial head fracture: a potentially complex injury. *Clin Orthop* 1993, 297:224–230.

2. Hotchkiss RN: Displaced fractures of the radial head: internal fixation or excision? *J Am Acad Orthop Surg* 1997, 5:1–10.

Diagnosis

History
Fall on an outstretched arm.
Elbow pain.
Inability to rotate forearm.

Physical findings
Diffuse swelling and elbow effusion.
Tenderness over proximal radius.
Pain on passive or active forearm rotation.

Imaging and laboratory studies
Radiographs: a true anteroposterior and lateral radiograph of the elbow is required. If the radial head is not ossified and a radial neck fracture is suspected, the diagnosis can be made with ultrasonography or arthrography of the elbow joint.

Complications
Loss of motion, specifically pronation and supination.
Premature closure of the physis.
Radial head overgrowth.
Avascular necrosis.
Neurologic injury.

Differential diagnosis
Nondisplaced lateral condyle fracture.
Nursemaid's elbow.

Etiology or pathophysiology
The injury usually occurs secondary to a fall on an outstretched arm. Because of the normal valgus-carrying angle, this transmits an axial load across the radial head. The resulting fracture can be metaphyseal or transphyseal (Salter-Harris Type I or II). Rarely, a Salter-Harris Type III or IV injury occurs with a shear through the radial head. A radial neck fracture can also occur during a posterior elbow dislocation (the proximal fragment is anteriorly displaced) or during the reduction of a posterior elbow dislocation (the proximal fragment is posteriorly displaced).

Epidemiology
Fractures of the radial neck account for 1% of children's fractures.

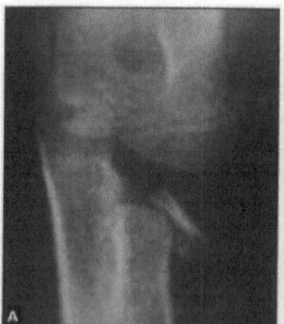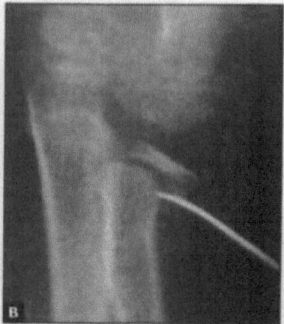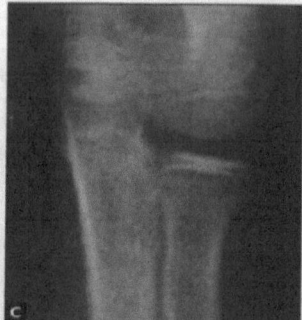

Figure 1. A, Displaced radial neck fracture. B, Percutaneous reduction done using no. 4 Penfield. C, Final reduction.

Treatment

Nonsurgical

Nondisplaced and minimally displaced fractures with up to 30° of angulation and 3 mm of translocation can be immobilized for about 10 days. Protected range of motion should then begin for another 2 to 3 weeks to prevent elbow stiffness. Many displaced fractures can be reduced under general anesthesia by closed reduction that involves applying longitudinal traction, valgus stress, and direct pressure over the displaced radial head. Image intensification is needed. A second method is to flex the elbow to 90° and place direct pressure over the radial head while forcefully pronating the forearm. Whatever technique is used, 50° to 60° of pronation and supination should be noted after the reduction.

Surgical

Open reduction is necessary if an acceptable reduction cannot be achieved via a closed method. Often, percutaneous reduction is possible by using a Steinmann pin or no. 4 Penfield as a skid (Fig. 1). Internal fixation is necessary only for reduced fractures that are not stable and is done to prevent redisplacement. One oblique bicortical pin usually suffices.

Treatment aims
To maintain full range of motion of the elbow and forearm.

Prognosis
Despite proper treatment, stiffness may occur at the site of many displaced radial neck fractures. The risk increases with associated injuries or need for operative intervention. The loss of motion is usually well tolerated.

Follow-up and management
After closed or open reduction, protected active range of motion is started as soon as possible, usually about 14 days after the procedure. Internal fixation is usually removed at about 2 to 3 weeks to begin early range of motion. Full activity can begin if radiographic evidence shows fracture healing.

Key references
1. Chambers HG, Wilkins KE: Fractures of the proximal radius. In *Fractures in Children.* Edited by Rockwood CA, Wilkins KE, Beaty JH. Philadelphia: Lippincott–Raven; 1996:586–613.

RHEUMATOID ARTHRITIS   J.D. Mabrey

Diagnosis

History
Keeping in mind the seven American College of Rheumatology (ACR) criteria (discussed below), the patient may report pain around one or several joints or systemic pain with no particular joint involvement. A family history of rheumatoid arthritis, systemic lupus erythematosus, or Reiter's syndrome may suggest a genetic component.

Physical findings
Affected joints may demonstrate increased warmth and swelling, painful motion, and flexion contracture. Rheumatoid nodules may be present over the dorsal aspect of the arm. Chest expansion is limited in patients with ankylosing spondylitis. In addition to the joints of the extremities, the temporomandibular, sternoclavicular, and sternomanubrial joints should be examined. Severely involved knees may be in extreme valgus (knock-knee). Heberden's nodes are noted about the distal interphalangeal joints of the hand, while Bouchard's nodes are noted about the proximal interphalangeal joints. The metacarpal phalangeal joints may demonstrate subluxation and ulnar drift.

The seven ACR criteria for rheumatoid arthritis are 1) morning stiffness in and around joints lasting at least 1 hour before maximal improvement; 2) soft tissue swelling or arthritis of three or more joint areas observed by a physician; 3) swelling or arthritis of the proximal interphalangeal, metacarpophalangeal, or wrist joints; 4) symmetric swelling or arthritis; 5) rheumatoid nodules; 6) the presence of rheumatoid factor; and 7) radiographic erosions or periarticular osteopenia in hand or wrist joints. For diagnosis rheumatoid arthritis, criteria 1 through 4 must have been present for at least 6 weeks, and a patient must have 4 of the 7 criteria for more than 6 weeks.

Imaging and laboratory studies
Plain radiographs of joints involved with rheumatoid arthritis may demonstrate periarticular soft tissue swelling, osteoporosis, loss of the subchondral bony plate, symmetrical joint space narrowing, and periarticular cysts.

Lateral flexion and extension radiographs of the cervical spine are essential to rule out subluxation of C1 on C2, measured as the distance between the anterior margin of the dens and the atlas. A distance of 3 mm or less is acceptable.

C-reactive protein: monitoring of inflammation.

Antinuclear antibodies: evaluating for systemic lupus erythematosus.

Rheumatoid factor: positive in 75% to 90% of patients with rheumatoid arthritis.

HLA-B27: strong association with spondyloarthropathies; 95% in ankylosing spondylitis; 80% in Reiter's syndrome.

Complications
Joint contracture and deformity.

Blindness from iridocyclitis (juvenile rheumatoid arthritis).

Loss of ambulation.

Osteoporosis.

Infection from surgical interventions.

Spinal cord injury from cervical subluxation.

Poor wound healing.

Compromised immune system and increased fracture risk from the use of steroids.

Differential diagnosis
Seronegative arthropathies.
Crystalline arthropathies.
Joint infection.
Lyme disease.

Etiology or pathophysiology
Rheumatoid arthritis is caused by activation and injury of synovial microvascular endothelial cells. Synovial lining then proliferates and forms microvilli that protrude into the joint space. Hypertrophic sublining synovial tissue composed of activated and invasive fibroblast-like cells invade and destroy periarticular bone and cartilage. The course of the disease is characterized by alternating periods of improvement and exacerbation; permanent remission occurs in only 10% to 15% of patients.

Epidemiology
Prevalence is estimated at 1% to 2% of the adult population and increases with age. Women are affected 2.5:1 over men, although the disease tends to be more severe in men. Juvenile rheumatoid arthritis is the most common form of arthritis in childhood, affecting up to 100,000 children.

Treatment

Nonsurgical

Nonpharmacologic
Patient education; occupational therapy; proper diet.

Pharmacologic
Steroids: in general, steroids should be avoided in the treatment of rheumatoid arthritis, except as bridging therapy between nonsteroidal anti-inflammatory drugs (NSAIDs) and disease-modifying antirheumatic drugs (DMARDs), for severe flares of the disease, and for intra-articular injections.

NSAIDs: these drugs are used as the initial agents in arresting the symptoms of inflammation. They include aspirin, salsalate, ibuprofen, and the new COX-2 inhibitors (eg, celecoxib).

DMARDs: these drugs should be initiated when arthritis no longer responds to NSAIDs. Most of these agents (except for methotrexate) require more than 8 weeks to become effective. In addition to methotrexate, this class includes hydroxy-chloroquine, azathioprine, and penicillamine.

Newest therapies: etanercept is a new tumor necrosis factor antagonist that is just entering the market and has demonstrated tremendous potential. Leflunomide is a new immunosuppressive that may be used with DMARDs. It is well tolerated and has few side effects.

Surgical
Cervical fusion for severe spine involvement.

Synovectomy of affected joints.

Fusion of certain joints—eg, wrist.

Total joint replacement: shoulder, elbow, hip, knee, and ankle.

Exercise and activity modification
Patients should participate in water therapy in pools of 83°F as approved by the Arthritis Foundation. Patients also should participate in motion exercises like swimming or cycling to maintain range of motion.

Treatment aims
To prevent the progression of joint destruction and improve functional disability.

Prognosis
Most patients must live with the disease their entire lives. Many end up with multiple joint replacements and may suffer side effects from various medications.

Follow-up and management
Constant monitoring of renal and hepatic function is essential if the patient is receiving multiple medications. Gastric ulcers are also a problem. Routine follow-up for total joint care is necessary to rule out infection or failure of the joint.

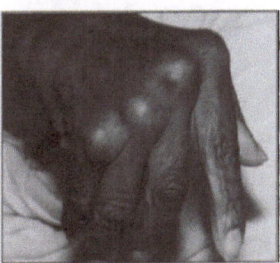

Figure 1. Right hand of a patient with long-standing rheumatoid arthritis. Note the ulnar deviation of the metacarpophalangeal (MCP) joints. Many patients' hands are functional despite this deformity, but others may require replacement of the MCPs with silastic implants.

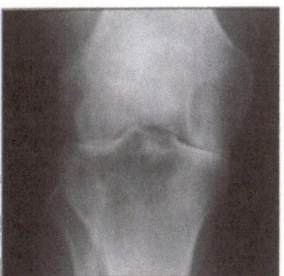

Figure 2. Anteroposterior (AP) plain radiograph of the knee of a patient with rheumatoid arthritis showing diffuse osteopenia, complete loss of the cartilage interval in both the medial and lateral aspects of the joint, and complete absence of any osteophytes.

Key references
1. Arnett FC, Edworthy SM, Bloch DA, et al.: The American Rheumatism Association 1987 revised criteria for the classification of rheumatoid arthritis. *Arthritis Rheum* 1988, 31:315–324.

2. Schumacher HR: *Primer on the Rheumatic Diseases* edn 10. Atlanta: The Arthritis Foundation; 1993.

3. Sculco TP: *Surgical Treatment of Rheumatoid Arthritis.* St. Louis: Mosby–Year Book; 1992.

P. Jacobs

Diagnosis

History
Night pain.

Pain in affected shoulder.

Decreased range of motion.

Difficulty with overhead activities and placing hand behind head.

With history of dislocation, increased risk for rotator cuff tears in patients aged more than 40 years.

Important to document sport or occupation if involved with injury.

Physical findings
Decreased range of motion.

Weakness (important to test rotator cuff muscles individually to assess strength).

Supraspinatus: isometric elevation of the arm held in 90° of elevation in the plane of the scapula in mild internal rotation.

Infraspinatus: isometric external rotation with arm at side in neutral rotation with the elbow flexed 90°.

Subscapularis: lift-off test; Napoleon sign.

Palpation: when proximal humerus is rotated under a finger placed over anterior acromion, defect in rotator cuff can often be palpated.

Instability.

Neurovascular examination: important to rule out cervical radicular symptoms.

Good neck examination, including testing of range of motion and Spurling's sign.

Laboratory and radiographic studies
Plain radiographs: anteroposterior, axillary lateral, and 30° caudal tilt (look for humeral head elevation, subacromial spur).

Arthrography: gold standard for many years.

Magnetic resonance imaging: 90% specific and sensitive (Fig. 1).

Ultrasonography: Highly technical and radiologist-dependent; in the proper hands, at least 90% sensitive and specific.

Complications
Failed cuff repair.

Failed acromioplasty.

Adhesions.

Persistent crepitus.

Recurrent rotator cuff tear.

Failed rehabilitation.

Differential diagnosis
Rotator cuff tendinitis.

Subacromial/subdeltoid bursitis.

Frozen shoulder/adhesive capsulitis.

Snapping scapula.

Glenohumeral arthritis.

Acromioclavicular arthritis.

Suprascapular neuropathy.

Cervical radicular symptoms.

Pancoast tumor.

Referred pain (eg, diaphragmatic pain).

Etiology or pathophysiology
Acute versus chronic.

Traumatic versus degenerative.

Macrotraumatic versus microtraumatic.

Important to determine partial- versus full-thickness tear.

Epidemiology
Cadaver studies have incidence of 5% to 20% with full-thickness tears.

Risk for rotator cuff tear and risk for associated rotator cuff tears in shoulder dislocations increase in persons more than 40 years of age.

Occupations or job positions associated with increased risk:
Ranching. Tree pruning. Fruit picking. Nursing. Carpenter. Painter.

Sports associated with increased risk for rotator cuff tears:
Overhead athlete (pitcher, quarterback). Tennis. Swimming. Skiing.

Treatment

Nonsurgical

Asymptomatic cuff tears: conservative treatment if needed (rotator cuff strengthening program).

Partial-thickness lesions:

Physical therapy: range of motion, stretching; when range of motion is regained, start rotator cuff strengthening program.

Nonsteroidal anti-inflammatory drugs.

Cold and hot therapy.

Ultrasound.

Full-thickness lesions:

Rest and time.

Physical therapy (stretching/range of motion/strengthening).

Nonsteroidal anti-inflammatory drugs.

Subacromial injection: only recommended if surgery is not an option.

Surgical

Partial-thickness lesions: if lesion is greater than 50% of cuff thickness, surgery may be indicated for debridement and repair, as is done for full-thickness rotator cuff tear.

Full-thickness lesions: open versus arthroscopic.

Acute tears: surgery decreases pain and improves function.

Chronic tears: in patients less than 60 years of age; failure of conservative treatment; documented rotator cuff tear (identified by arthrography, magnetic resonance imaging, ultrasonography); full passive range of motion; ability of patient to comprehend and cooperate with rehabilitation.

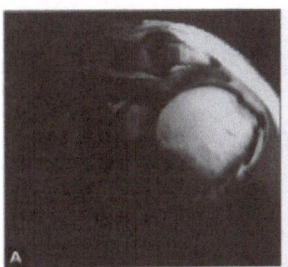 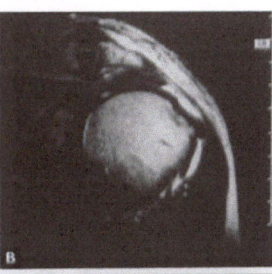

Figure 1. A and B, Magnetic resonance images of rotator cuff tears.

Treatment aims
To relieve pain.
To restore function (range of motion and strength).

Prognosis
Results are excellent to good in 75% to 80% of patients.

Follow-up and rehabilitation
Nonsurgical
Range of motion should be reestablished first, then progress to strengthening program.
Surgical
No driving for 4 to 6 weeks.
0 to 6 weeks: pendulums, passive range of motion (forward flexion and external rotation).
6 weeks to 6 months: rotator cuff strengthening program.
Full release by 6 months.

Key references
1. Bigliani LU, Post M, Flatow EL, et al.: The Shoulder: Operative Technique. Baltimore: Williams & Wilkins; 1998:133–165.
2. Cofield RH: Current concepts review: rotator cuff disease of the shoulder. J Bone Joint Surg [Am] 1985, 67:974–979.
3. Matsen FA, Arntz CT, Lippitt SB: Rotator cuff. In The Shoulder edn 5. Edited by Rockwood CA, Matsen FA. Philadelphia: WB Saunders; 1998:755–839.
4. Matsen FA III, Lippitt SB, Sidles JA, et al.: Practical Evaluation and Management of the Shoulder. Philadelphia: WB Saunders; 1994:1–242.

Diagnosis

History
Most scaphoid fractures occur when excessive force is applied to the wrist while the wrist is dorsiflexed. Associated periscaphoid injuries can occur from the force applied, depending on the relative position of the wrist at the moment of fracture.

Physical findings
Well-localized tenderness to palpation in the anatomic snuffbox is the hallmark sign of a scaphoid fracture. With an isolated fracture, signs of neurovascular compromise are rare. Such findings are more suggestive of greater carpal injury.

Imaging and laboratory studies
Most fractures can be detected with orthogonal radiographs of the wrist (Fig. 1). Additional flexion, extension, radial, and ulnar deviation films should allow the detection of 90% of scaphoid fractures. A scaphoid fracture that initially presents with "normal" radiographs will show radiographic changes within 3 weeks of injury. Bone scanning, computed tomography, and magnetic resonance imaging are rarely necessary to diagnose a scaphoid fracture during these 3 weeks.

Complications
The major complication is nonunion of the fracture caused by insufficient fracture immobilization and poor vascularity at the fracture site. Persistent nonunion can lead to periscaphoid instability, with resultant posttraumatic wrist arthritis.

Differential diagnosis
The major injuries that should be differentiated from a scaphoid fracture include a distal radius fracture, a lunate fracture, and a scapholunate dissociation. All occur in the same region of the wrist with localized tenderness. Scrutiny of the radiographs should allow for differentiation.

Etiology or pathophysiology
Most scaphoid fractures occur from a fall onto the outstretched hand.

Epidemiology
Scaphoid fractures are less common than distal radius fractures and are more likely to occur in men. These fractures generally occur in persons younger than those who sustain distal radius fractures.

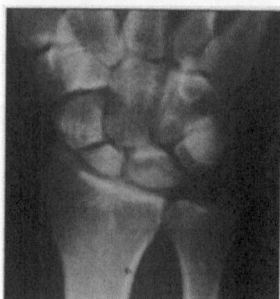

Figure 1. Radiograph of a scaphoid fracture.

Treatment

Nonsurgical
The most common treatment of an acute injury involves a cast that immobilizes the wrist and thumb (ie, thumb spica cast). Some authorities use a below-elbow cast; others favor an above-elbow case. Adjuncts to casting have involved both electrical and ultrasonographic stimulation to enhance fracture healing.

Surgical
The initial treatment of an acute scaphoid fracture is usually nonoperative because fracture displacement or angulation is minimal. Displaced fractures are often associated with further carpal instability. In these cases, open fracture reduction with wire or screw fixation of the scaphoid may be necessary to stabilize the wrist and optimize conditions for fracture healing. Nonunion of a scaphoid fracture, however, is commonly treated surgically with exposure of the nonunion, scaphoid fixation, and bone grafting.

Exercise and activity modification
Cessation of smoking during fracture treatment is strongly suggested.

Treatment aims
Solid fracture union and full, painless wrist function are the goals of treatment.

Prognosis
Average healing time appears to be associated with fracture location. The more distal the fracture, the shorter the healing time. Tuberosity fractures may heal as quickly as 1 month after injury; proximal fifth fractures may take as long as 5 months. Similarly, increased fracture obliquity portends slower healing.

Follow-up and management
Routine periodic clinical and radiographic follow-up is important for assessment of fracture healing. Once it becomes apparent that fracture healing has slowed or stopped, operative treatment is generally used to promote fracture union. Rigid fixation of the unhealed fracture with or without bone graft is undertaken to change the mechanical and biologic environment at the site of osseous discontinuity.

Key references
1. Barton NJ: Twenty questions about scaphoid fractures. *J Hand Surg* 1992, 17B:289–310.
2. Russe O: Fracture of the carpal navicular. *J Bone Joint Surg* 1960, 42A:759–768.
3. Watson HK, Ashmead D IV, Makhlouf MV: Examination of the scaphoid. *J Hand Surg* 1988, 13A:657–660.

J.R. Warman

Diagnosis

History
Back pain that worsens with activity, sitting, and standing and is greater during periods of increased growth.

Symptoms that improve with skeletal maturity.

Patients self-report of poor body image.

Physical findings
When bending forward and viewed laterally, patients with thoracic Scheuermann's disease exhibit a sharp kyphos. Unlike postural kyphosis, the curve is stiff and cannot be voluntarily straightened. There may be some local tenderness. A thorough neurologic examination should be performed.

Imaging and laboratory studies
Radiographs: Standing anteroposterior and lateral views are necessary to evaluate the spine. Radiographic criteria for thoracic Scheuermann's disease is 5° of wedging seen on at least three successive vertebra (Fig. 1). Irregularity of the end plates, narrowing of the disk space, and Schmorl's nodes are also present. Wedging is not noted in lumbar Scheuermann's disease, in which lumbar lordosis is maintained. Flexibility of the thoracic kyphos is determined by a supine cross-table radiograph with a soft bolster at the apex of the deformity.

Complications
Spondylolysis.

Mild scoliosis.

Disk herniations or mechanical compression impinging on the spinal cord (rare).

Differential diagnosis
Postural kyphosis
When these patients bend forward, no acute gibbus or kyphos is noted. The curve may also be actively or passively fully correctable.

Congenital kyphosis
May be due to a failure of formation or of segmentation of the vertebral body. These types of kyphosis are progressive and can cause neurologic compromise. Spinal cord, renal, cardiac, and other anomalies may be present.

Etiology or pathophysiology
It is believed the deformity is caused by a growth disturbance of the vertebral body end plates. This may be mechanical in nature, following Wolff's law, as is suggested by the success of bracing in some patients.

The high familial predilection suggests a genetic component.

Histologic examination shows disorganized enchondral ossification of the vertebral growth plate.

Epidemiology
The incidence ranges from 0.5% to 10% in the general population.

There is a male preponderance.

Scheuermann's disease usually occurs during puberty.

Thoracic Scheuermann's disease is typical.

Atypical Scheuermann's disease occurs in the thoracolumbar and lumbar spine.

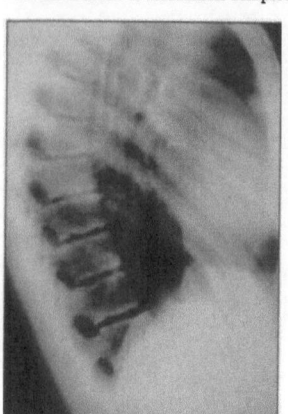

Figure 1. Wedging of vertebral bodies, narrowing of the disk space, and irregular end plates on radiograph of a patient with Scheuermann's disease.

Treatment

Nonsurgical

Smaller, nonprogressive curves may be observed by serial radiographs at 4- to 6-month intervals. Skeletally immature patients with progressive curves may be treated with a hyperextension brace during waking hours. Bracing is weaned and discontinued when skeletal maturity is reached. The deformity often reverses with such treatment. Treatment of stiffer curves may begin with a series of casts to loosen the curve before bracing. A thoracic lumbar sacral orthosis is used to treat the symptoms of lumbar Scheuermann's disease when present.

Surgical

Surgery is recommended for progressive kyphosis when bracing is unsuccessful or for larger curves in skeletally mature patients. Curves correctable to 50° may be treated with posterior instrumentation and fusion, whereas larger, stiffer curves require anterior release and fusion before the posterior surgery. Surgical complications include spinal cord injury, pseudoarthrosis, failure of the hardware, and pull-out of the instrumentation.

Treatment aims

For thoracic Scheuermann's disease, to prevent further progression of the kyphotic deformity or to correct the deformity; for lumbar Scheuermann's disease, to relieve symptoms.

Prognosis

The natural history of thoracic Scheuermann's disease is for most rapid progression during the adolescent growth spurt. Pulmonary function is not compromised until the curve surpasses 100°. It is not known whether the kyphosis progresses during adulthood. No significant clinical or functional problems have been noted in adults, but these patients do have mild increased back pain.

Key references

1. Ascani E, LaRosa G: Scheuermann's kyphosis. In *The Pediatric Spine: Principles and Practice.* Edited by Weinstein SL. New York: Raven Press; 1994:557–584.

2. Warner WC: Kyphosis. In *Lovell and Winter's Pediatric Orthopedics.* Edited by Morrissy RT, Weinstein SL. Philadelphia: Lippincott–Raven; 1996:689–699.

Diagnosis

History

Ill-fitting clothing, shoulder drop, curving spine, or a rib hump are signs of idiopathic scoliosis. Patients with neurogenic scoliosis may also have weakness, loss of balance, joint contracture, and urinary or fecal incontinence. Back pain is rare with idiopathic scoliosis but may be present in scoliosis caused by such lesions as spinal cord tumor. Patients with severe scoliosis may have respiratory insufficiency.

Physical findings

The earliest sign is prominence of the paravetebral muscles on the convex side of the curve, seen when the patient bends over at the waist. This occurs because the spine not only curves but also rotates into the convexity of the curve, elevating lumbar muscles or ribs (Fig. 1). The shoulder may be depressed, with truncal shift and head balance decompensation. Neurologic signs are present in scoliosis because of cerebral palsy, muscular dystrophy, and other neurologic conditions and often include muscle weakness, spasticity, abnormal deep tendon reflexes, and ankle clonus. In scoliosis due to spinal cord tumor, abnormal abdominal reflexes and tight hamstrings may be present.

Imaging and laboratory studies

A standing anteroposterior and lateral radiograph of the entire spine is taken to assess location and magnitude of the curve and to detect congenital scoliosis abnormalities such as hemivertebrae, fused vertebrae, or unilateral unsegmented bars (Fig. 2). The Cobb angle is used to measure curves: lines are placed on the endplates of the end vertebrae at the proximal and distal end of the curve; lines perpendicular to those lines inscribe the angle of the curve. A Cobb angle greater than 10° is defined as scoliosis (Fig. 3). An increase in the Cobb angle by 5° or more defines the scoliosis as a progressive curve. Rotation of the vertebrae is assessed by pedicle position. Skeletal maturity is estimated by the extent of ossification of the iliac apophysis (ie, the Risser sign). Other congenital lesions associated with scoliosis include diastematomyelia and posterior element dysraphism. Intradural spinal cord tumor may cause medial flattening of the pedicles and increased interpedicular distance. Vertebral tumors may obliterate the pedicles or erode vertebral bodies. Computed tomography scans can be done to assess congenital deformity of the spine and bony tumors. Magnetic resonance imaging scans are useful for ruling out spinal cord cysts and tumors.

Complications

May affect pulmonary function. At 60° or greater, exercise tolerance is affected, and from 90° to 110°, cor pulmonale may develop.

Differential diagnosis

Congenital scoliosis. Neurogenic scoliosis due to cerebral palsy or muscular dystrophy. Spinal cord tumor. Osteoid osteoma. Osteomyelitis of the spine. Spinal cord syrinx. Functional scoliosis.

Etiology

Eighty percent of cases are idiopathic. These cases are usually found in female adolescents with thoracic scoliosis convex to the right. In the remaining cases, the scoliosis has an identifiable cause, such as neurogenic disease, primary vertebral malformation, or secondary lesions (eg, spinal cord tumor). Conditions such as mechanical back pain or splinting with pneumonia can produce a functional scoliosis that is notable because the vertebrae is not rotated on radiography.

Epidemiology

Incidence ranges from 1.5% to 3% of growing children.

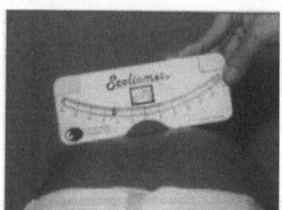

Figure 1. Scoliosis is clinically assessed with a scoliometer measuring rotation of the torso.

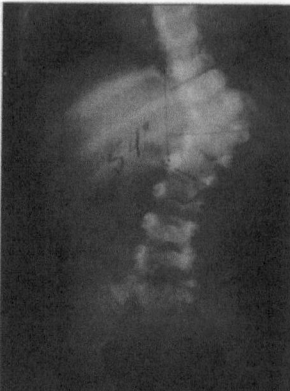

Figure 2. A young patient with congenital scoliosis resulting from hemivertebra.

Treatment

Nonsurgical

Curves under 20°: observation.

Curves that are 20° to 40°, are progressive, and occur in a growing child: brace.

Curves that are greater than 40° and are progressive: posterior spinal fusion dual-rod with instrumentation.

Surgical

For very severe curves, both anterior and posterior spine fusion may be necessary. Neurogenic curves require long fusions with Luque instrumentation. Congenital curves usually undergo in situ posterior convex arthrodesis without instrumentation; anterior epiphysiodesis is added for some curves. Spinal cord tumors, syrinx, or tethered cord first require neurosurgical treatment (Fig. 4), with later spine fusion as indicated. A severe rib hump can be treated with thoracoplasty. If possible, fusion is done in children no younger than 10 years of age to minimize growth inhibition.

Treatment aims

To arrest the progression of the curve, correct it as much as possible, and stabilize it with surgery if necessary. To restore balance and symmetry of the torso. To maintain normal pulmonary function.

Prognosis

Prognosis is excellent if treatment begins before curves become severe.

Follow-up and management

Follow-up visits should be held at least every 6 months, with physical examination and a posteroanterior standing radiograph of the entire spine. Worrisome curves should be followed up every 3 months. Patients wearing a brace undergo radiography out of the brace. Patients who develop progressive curves despite bracing will need spinal fusion. Yearly follow-up is needed until patients reach skeletal maturity.

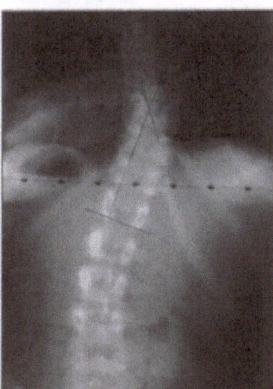

Figure 3. The Cobb angle is marked on this typical example of idiopathic, adolescent scoliosis. The curve's apex is toward the right and is thoracic in location.

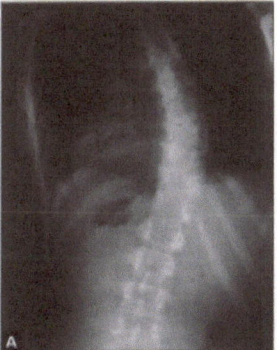
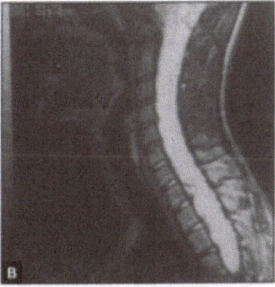

Figure 4. A, Right thoracic curve in an adolescent male. Medial thinning of the pedicles is seen in the midthoracic spine. A subtle hip flexor weakness was seen on a physical examination. B, MRI of the entire spine revealed a holocord astrocytoma. The patient was treated with laminectomy and resection of the tumor.

Key references

1. King HA, Moe JH, Bradford DS, et al.: The selection of fusion levels in thoracic idiopathic scoliosis. *J Bone Joint Surg [Am]* 1983, 65:1302.

2. Weinstein SL, Zavala D, Ponsetti IV: Idiopathic scoliosis: long term follow-up and prognosis in untreated patients. *J Bone Joint Surg [Am]* 1981, 63:701.

3. Winter RB: Convex anterior and posterior hemiarthrodesis and hemiepiphysiodesis in young children with progressive congenital scoliosis. *J Pediatr Orthop* 1981, 1:361.

Diagnosis

History

Patients with septic arthritis have acute onset of pain in the joint with swelling. A limp or complete inability to bear weight on the affected side is common in lower-extremity septic arthritis. Fever and malaise are often present.

Physical findings

Features include a tender joint with effusion, pain with motion, and surrounding muscle spasm. The joint position is one of maximum volume to decrease painful pressure: the hip is held in abduction, flexion, and external rotation; the knee and elbow are held in flexion; the ankle is held in neutral; the shoulder is held in mild abduction. Mild gentle rotation of the joint results in greater muscle spasm.

Imaging and laboratory studies

Anteroposterior and lateral radiographs are taken to rule out osteomyelitis. In septic arthritis, usually only deep soft tissue edema is seen, but lateral joint subluxation may be present in the hip and the shoulder. Technetium bone scans are generally negative in septic arthritis but can be used to detect early associated osteomyelitis. Ultrasonography is useful for detecting hip joint effusions.

Laboratory studies should include a complete blood count with erythrocyte sedimentation rate, blood cultures, and measurement of C-reactive protein level. An elevated leukocyte count with a shift to the left, increased sedimentation rate, and elevated C-reactive protein level suggest active infection. All suspected septic joints should undergo aspiration under sterile conditions; if the shoulder or hip is affected, general anesthesia is required for successful aspiration. All aspirates should undergo routine aerobic and anaerobic culture and Gram stain, and part of the specimen should be inoculated into blood culture bottles for higher rate of organism identification. It is also important to measure protein and glucose levels and the leukocyte count of the joint fluid. Some have found patients with septic arthritis have high protein levels and low glucose levels. A leukocyte cell count greater than 80,000 cells/mm^3, with polymorphonuclear cells greater than 75%, is seen in septic arthritis.

Complications

Articular cartilage damage, progressing to early degenerative joint disease, can occur with septic arthritis. The hip in the growing child can also undergo avascular necrosis, causing severe growth disturbance.

Differential diagnosis
Transient synovitis of the hip.
Traumatic synovitis.
Juvenile rheumatoid arthritis.
Rheumatic fever.
Hemophilic arthropathy.
Osteomyelitis.
Leukemia cell joint infiltrates.

Etiology
A transient bacteremia probably seeds the joint, and clinical infection occurs when a certain threshold of bacteria is reached. The most common organism found depends on the age of the patient:
Neonate: *Staphylococcus aureus*, group B streptococci, enteric bacilli.
1 month to 3 years: *Haemophilus influenzae* (if the patient is not vaccinated), *S. aureus*, group A and B streptococci, gram-negative bacilli.
Older than 3 years: *S. aureus*, hemolytic streptococci, gram-negative bacilli.

Epidemiology
In the 1970s, *H. influenzae* type B had become the most common cause of septic arthritis in young children. However, because of use of a new vaccine in the 1990s, this organism is now less common. This is important because 30% of patients with *H. influenzae* septic arthritis have concurrent meningitis.

Treatment

If joint aspiration obtains relatively clear fluid, the patient receives intravenous therapy with a broad-spectrum antibiotic while cultures are pending. If cultures prove to be positive, arthrotomy is done (Fig. 1). If the fluid is cloudy, a joint arthrotomy is performed immediately to augment antibiotic coverage. In infants and children up to age 4 years, *S. aureus* is most likely the organism if the patient has been vaccinated for *H. influenzae*; in patients who have not been vaccinated, *H. influenzae* is the most likely organism. In both groups, intravenous cefuroxime (100 to 150 mg/kg of body weight per day, administered every 8 hours) is a good choice. In older patients, intravenous oxacillin (150 mg/kg/d, administered every 6 hours), methicillin (150 mg/k/d, administered every 6 hours), or cefazolin (100 mg/k/d, administered 8 hours) is a good choice for initial coverage. If later cultures are positive, then the antibiotic is changed to one specific for that organism. However, 20% to 60% of cases of septic arthritis are culture-negative, and patients must continue to be treated with broad-spectrum antibiotics. While receiving intravenous antibiotics in the hospital, patients are monitored for decreased tenderness and swelling of the joint, defervescence, return of appetite, and ability to use the extremity normally. With successful treatment, levels of C-reactive protein decrease within days, but sedimentation rates tend to stay elevated for weeks.

Once improvement is seen clinically, discharge to outpatient status is considered. Conversion to oral antibiotics is possible if the following criteria are satisfied: the organism is isolated and an oral antibiotic is available for its treatment, bactericidal levels of oral antibiotics to the isolated organism are obtained, the patient can tolerate the antibiotic, and there is reasonable assurance that the family will comply to complete a course of treatment. The choice of oral antibiotics depend on culture results. Antibiotic treatment can last from 3 weeks for mild cases to 6 weeks for more severe disease. Serial determinations of C-reactive protein levels and sedimentation rate assist decisions about length of treatment.

Some physicians consider serial needle aspirations to be adequate for joint drainage in septic arthritis. With needle aspiration, however, joint loculations are difficult to remove, and aspiration of fluid from the hip joint is especially difficult. Arthrotomy is the option preferred by most orthopedists.

Treatment aims
To identify the site of septic arthritis.
To identify the causative organism.
To treat septic arthritis with appropriate antibiotics and surgery when necessary.
To restore the child's normal function.

Prognosis
Prognosis is excellent with prompt treatment. If septic arthritis of the hip is not treated within 4 days of onset, prognosis is guarded and avascular necrosis may develop.

Follow-up and management
The patient should be followed weekly until wounds are healed and painless active range of motion of the joint is achieved. Until skeletal maturity is reached, yearly follow-up is needed with patients who did not receive prompt treatment, especially those with hip infection.

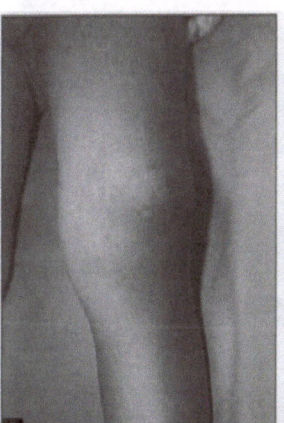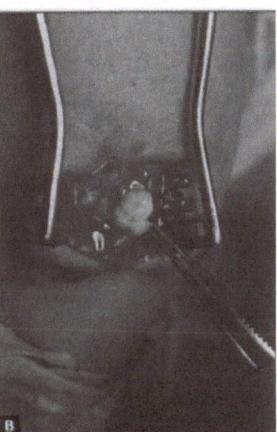

Figure 1. A, A young patient with septic arthritis of the knee with swelling and erythema of the joint resulting in painful spasm with attempted motion. B, Loculations of purulent material are removed during arthrotomy of the knee.

Key references
1. Morrissy RT: Bone and joint sepsis in children. *Instructional Course Lectures* vol 31. Rosemont, IL: American Academy of Orthopaedic Surgeons; 1982:49.

Diagnosis

History

Most patients with seronegative spondyloarthropathy with spinal symptoms have ankylosing spondylitis (AS). A small percentage of patients with psoriatic arthropathy, spondyloarthropathy associated with inflammatory bowel disease (IBD), or reactive arthropathy secondary to Reiter's syndrome may also have pain. Patients with AS usually have a history of insidious onset of low back pain (LBP) and stiffness in the second or third decade of life. Pain varies in location from the gluteal region to the lumbar or thoracic spine. Pain in the buttocks with radiation to the legs is common and can be confused with sciatica; however, pain from AS seldom radiates below the knee. Symptoms usually worsen in the morning and improve with exercise, which distinguishes AS from mechanical back pain that is worse with activity but improves with rest. Patients often complain of night pain and frequent sleep interruptions. Patients with chronic involvement may develop lumbar, thoracic, and cervical kyphosis with cephalad progression. With time, patients develop a progressive kyphosis with limited cervical and thoracic extension resulting in a stooped posture. Back and neck pain may eventually improve (past ankylosis), with spinal deformity becoming the major complaint.

Physical findings

Patients with no history of spondyloarthropathy must be evaluated for psoriasis, IBD, or Reiter's syndrome. All AS patients will have spine involvement, compared with < 20% of those with other seronegative spondyloarthropathies. Early in the course of AS, physical examination is less useful. With disease progression, the measurement of cervical rotation, chest expansion, and finger-to-floor distance becomes more sensitive. Laboratory tests have limited value. Elevation of erythrocyte sedimentation rate and C-reactive protein is common but correlates poorly with clinical progression of the disease. AS is strongly associated with the class 1 antigen HLA-B27, which is common in 80% to 98% of affected white patients compared with only 8% of the general population. Commonly used criteria for diagnosing AS include LBP and stiffness for > 3 months that is not relieved with rest; pain and stiffness of the thoracic region; limited motion in the lumbar spine; limited chest expansion; and history or evidence of neuritis.

Imaging and laboratory studies

Radiographs are the most specific test for AS. Radiographic evidence of sacroileitis occurs early and is usually bilateral and symmetric. Spinal changes generally develop from the sacrum to the cervical spine with frequent "skip lesions." Anterior squaring of the vertebrae and sclerosis at disk insertions are common early in the disease. Linear radiodensities that connect adjacent vertebrae, called *syndesmophytes*, result from ossification of the annulus fibrosus and occur later; calcification of the interspinous and supraspinous ligaments also occurs later. A single anteroposterior pelvic radiograph to detect sacroiliac joint changes may be useful. CT is more sensitive than conventional radiography for early detection; magnetic resonance imaging (MRI) is more sensitive for detection of inflammatory changes. There is little evidence that early diagnosis of AS changes treatment or outcome; therefore, cost-effectiveness becomes an issue.

Complications

Progressive spinal deformity with decreased quality of life is a major complication. Spinal fracture is an uncommon but serious complication in advanced disease. Fractures often occur at the C5 and C6 levels but can involve any spinal segment; they may often be caused by minimal trauma due to decreased flexibility of the ankylosed spine. Spondylodiskitis, which can occur in advanced AS, consists of focal activity-related pain accompanied by erosive sclerotic lesions in adjacent vertebral bodies. It is not clear whether this is an inflammatory process or the result of trauma, but it appears similar to infectious diskitis or pseudarthrosis on radiographs. Anterior atlantoaxial subluxation has also been described. Patients with long-standing disease may develop insidious cauda equina syndrome with sensory loss, lower extremity weakness, bowel and bladder dysfunction, and impotence.

Differential diagnosis

Degenerative lumbar disk disease, rheumatoid arthritis, Reiter's syndrome, IBD, psoriatic arthropathy, musculoskeletal back pain, compression fracture, Paget's disease.

Etiology or pathophysiology

Patients with a history of psoriasis or Reiter's syndrome have less severe spinal involvement (< 20% of cases). Predominant etiology of LBP in these patients is sacroileitis. Patients with IBD have spondyloarthropathy in approximately 20% of cases; however, involvement of the axial spine is radiographically indistinguishable from AS. Sacroileitis associated with AS and IBD is bilateral and symmetric and syndesmophyte development is in cephalad progression; psoriatic or Reiter's spondyloarthropathy is unilateral and asymmetric and the syndesmophyte is randomly distributed. Characteristic pathology of AS involves inflammation, bony erosions, and ankylosis. Inflammation is lymphocytic; target tissues include joints and entheses. In the axial skeleton, the sacroiliac, apophyseal, and costovertebral joints are involved and eventually become ankylosed. Inflammation of the entheses occurs due to involvement of the annulus fibrosus junction and vertebral end plates. This leads to cortical erosion and characteristic squaring of vertebral bodies. Progressive annular ossification leads to bridging syndesmophytes with classic "bamboo spine." The role of HLA-B27 is unknown. It may be a receptor for an inciting antigen such as a virus, or AS may be incited by infections and environmental agents in patients made susceptible by the HLA-B27 locus. Extraspinal involvement is common and frequently involves peripheral arthritis. Hip involvement is common and often bilateral. Other sites include the shoulder, knee, wrist, metacarpophalangeal and metatarsophalangeal joints, ischial tuberosity, iliac crest, epicondyles of the elbows and shoulders, plantar fascia insertions, Achilles tendon, and ocular, cardiac, and pulmonary systems. Anterior uveitis occurs in 20% to 25% of patients.

Epidemiology

Patients between 15 and 50 years of age. Incidence in the U.S. is 67 to 197 cases per 100,000. The ratio of males to females varies between 1:1 and 4:1. Prevalence in women may be underestimated because disease is less severe and women are less likely to obtain a pelvic radiograph.

Treatment

Nonsurgical

The primary objectives of treating AS are to maintain proper posture and improve joint mobility. This is achieved with frequent exercise and physical therapy. Use of nonsteroidal anti-inflammatory drugs (NSAIDs) is helpful to minimize pain and stiffness and allow more comfortable physical therapy. Exercise programs are used for strengthening the back extensor muscles and maintaining spine, hip, and shoulder motion. Instituting exercise early in the course of the disease has been shown to have a strong correlation with improved function in patients who ultimately develop severe disease and ankylosis. Although exercise cannot prevent ankylosis, it can help to maintain a more functional upright posture. NSAIDs are the mainstay of medical management for AS. Corticosteroids have no proven value and their long-term use poses serious risks including osteoporosis. Occasional injections of corticosteroids in inflamed joints may help relieve symptomatic joint involvement. Gold, D-penicillamine, antimalarial drugs, and azothiaprine have been tested and shown to be of no value. Some trial studies with sulfasalazine have shown reductions in symptoms, but other studies have shown no differences in symptoms compared with placebo-treated groups. Cyclophosphamide and methyltrexate have been reported to improve symptoms but are still experimental.

Surgical

Surgical treatment is reserved for patients with severe deformity. Closing wedge extension osteotomies of the cervical and lumbar spine are the primary methods. Extension osteotomies of the lumbar spine have proved very successful, with an 88% patient satisfaction rate reported in one study. Currently, single level closing wedge osteotomy with instrumentation is the preferred method of treatment for patients with severe kyphoctic deformities and ankylosed spines.

Treatment aims

To maintain proper upright posture and joint mobility. Both nonsurgical and surgical methods of treatment are aimed at providing patients with a more functional and comfortable quality of life.

Prognosis

Long-term prognosis for patients with AS is directly dependent on the severity of the disease. Mild to moderate cases can be managed successfully with NSAIDs and physical therapy to achieve an adequate functional lifestyle for the patients. Patients with more severe disease with progressive ankylosis and spinal deformity have a poor prognosis for a functional quality of life.

Key references

1. Frymoyer JW: *The Adult Spine: Principles and Practice* edn 2. Philadelphia: Lippincott Raven, 1997:803–810.

2. Inflammatory arthritis of the spine: spondyloarthopathy. In *Orthopaedic Knowledge Update 6*. Edited by Arendt EA. Rosemont, IL: American Orthopaedic Society for Sports Medicine; 1999:685–690.

3. Simmons EH: Flexion deformities of the neck and ankylosing spondylitis. *J Bone Joint Surg* 1969, 51B:193–200.

4. Simmons EH: Kyphotic deformity of the spine and ankylosing spondylitis. *Clin Orthop* 1977, 128:65–77.

Diagnosis

History

Patients with slipped capital femoral epiphysis (SCFE) present with an external rotation limp. Pain is felt in the hip or thigh, but sometimes only the knee is painful through referral by the sensory branches of the obturator nerve. The latter presentation can easily lead to misdiagnosis. Presentation is described by four groups: 1) preslip SCFE, associated with a painful limp, mild limitation of hip motion, and normal radiographs; 2) acute SCFE, associated with severe pain of less than 3 weeks' duration, inability to bear weight, marked muscle spasm, and radiographs showing epiphyseal displacement with no signs of bony remodeling of the femoral neck; 3) chronic SCFE, associated with intermittent pain of greater than 3 weeks' duration, painful ambulation, limited hip motion, and epiphyseal slippage with femoral neck remodeling seen on radiography; and 4) acute or chronic SCFE associated with symptoms of a chronic slip, acute increase in pain and hip stiffness, and radiographs showing an acute epiphyseal displacement superimposed on femoral neck changes of a chronic slip. Loder *et al.* classified slips as unstable if the patient cannot bear weight on the affected side, regardless of duration of symptoms, and as stable if weight bearing is possible.

Physical findings

The affected hip is held in external rotation, and passive internal rotation is often impossible because of pain. Patients often have tenderness over the hip. All hip maneuvers must be gentle because vigorous motion of the hip may inadvertently worsen the slip or cause reduction of the femoral head with later complications. The presence of Percy's sign is pathognomonic of SCFE (Fig. 1): when the patient is sitting, the affected hip must be externally rotated for comfort, forcing the ipsilateral leg below the flexed knee into medial deviation.

Imaging and laboratory studies

SCFE is suspected if the epiphyseal plate is widened on radiographs. Klein's line (Fig. 2) is drawn along the superior border of the femoral neck extending into the femoral head; if the superior border of the femoral head is below this line, then SCFE is probable. Next, a careful "surgical lateral" radiograph of the hip is taken to detect posterior displacement of the femoral head on the neck. Frog-leg lateral radiographs of the hip are to be avoided because this position may further displace the slip. The maximum displacement of the epiphysis on the neck is graded: a minimal slip is less than one third the width of the femoral neck, a moderate slip is one third to one half the width of the femoral neck, and a severe slip is greater than one half the width of the femoral neck.

Complications

Untreated SCFE can progress, resulting in further displacement of the capital femoral epiphysis with worsening of limp and external rotation deformity of the hip. Avascular necrosis of the hip may also occur, but this is more likely in treated hips. In various series, patients treated by spica cast immobilization have a slip recurrence rate of 3% to 18%; avascular necrosis of the femoral head occurs in 7% of patients; skin ulcers occurred in 16%; and chondrolysis occurred in 19% to 67%. Only 4.6% of patients treated with in situ fixation by a single pin have pin-related complications compared with 36% of those treated with multiple pins. Attempted reduction of the slippage to improve position may result in rates of avascular necrosis of the hip as high as 31%, whereas in situ fixation without reduction is associated with a rate of 6%.

Differential diagnosis

Subcapital hip fracture, stress fracture of the hip, septic arthritis of the hip, osteoid osteoma of the femoral neck, or chondrolysis of the hip.

Etiology or pathophysiology

Almost all cases have an unknown cause, although most authors agree that the physeal plate is weakened and subject to abnormally high shear stress. Because most cases occur during adolescent growth spurt, hormonal factors are probably involved in alteration of physeal strength; however, no definitive relationship has been demonstrated. Incidence is increased in patients with endocrine disorders such as hypothyroidism, renal osteodystrophy, hypogonadal disease, and panhypopituitarism and in patients receiving growth hormone therapy.

Epidemiology

Incidence in the general population is 2/100,000. Black persons have a somewhat higher incidence. Male-to-female ratio is 2.4:1; boys present at an average age of 13.5 years (range, 10 to 16 years), and girls present at the average age of 11.5 (range, 10 to 14 years). Obesity is a risk factor. Skeletal age is delayed in most patients. The left hip is affected twice as often as the right, and bilateral SCFE is seen in 25% of cases. Half of the latter patients have bilateral disease at presentation; in the other half, the other slip usually develops within 18 months. Bilateral SCFE has been reported in 100% of patients with hypothyroid disease.

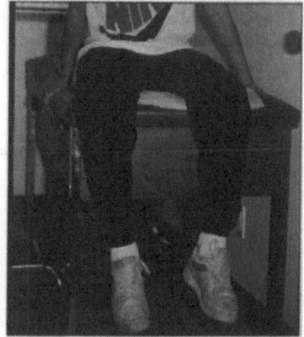

Figure 1. This patient with slipped capital femoral epiphysis of the right hip has Percy's sign. When the patient is seated the right hip is mildly rotated externally, turning the ipsilateral ankle toward the mid-line.

Treatment

The treatment for SCFE is in situ stabilization of the capital femoral epiphysis with a single cannulated screw into the femoral neck (Fig. 2). The technique can be done percutaneously under C-arm control unless the patient is morbidly obese. In such cases, open fixation through a lateral approach is used. For more severe slips, the screw is started into the anterior neck to approach the center of the head perpendicular to the physis. Screw penetration of the head is ruled out through range of motion of the hip under the C-arm.

Immobilization by a bilateral hip spica cast has been used by some authors, but most orthopedists do not use the technique because 1) patients find it hard to tolerate, 2) slips can continue to progress even during casting, 3) the complication rate is high, and 4) the approach is restricted to patients with minimal growth remaining. In very young patients for whom there is concern that crossing the hip epiphyseal plate with a threaded screw will arrest growth, either multiple smooth Kirschner wires or specially made proximal smooth shank screws can be used to stabilize the slip while permitting growth of the hip. In minimally displaced SCFE caused by untreated renal osteodystrophy, medical treatment includes close observation of the hip, with radiographs to document stabilization of the hip through improvement in the growth plate appearance. Surgical treatment for such cases is reserved for hips that continue to slip despite treatment. Late deformity in mature hips can be treated with proximal femoral osteotomies.

Treatment aims
To stabilize the epiphysis to the femoral neck, relieve pain, and prevent further deformity.
To induce closure of the unstable femoral physis.

Prognosis
Prognosis is excellent for stable hips in which SCFE is treated with in situ cannulated screw fixation. Unstable hips with SCFE treated by screw fixation have a higher rate of avascular necrosis.

Follow-up and management
Follow-up anteroposterior and lateral radiography of the hip 1 month after surgery to assess loosening of the screw or further progression of the slip. Visits should then be held every 3 months. Use crutches for partial weight bearing only on the operative side until radiographic evidence shows fusion of the epiphyseal plate. Activities can be gradually advanced at that point. If the patient desires, the screws can be removed 1 year after insertion. Radiographs should be obtained of hips with any signs or symptoms of contralateral SCFE.

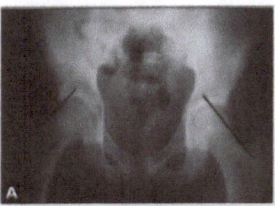
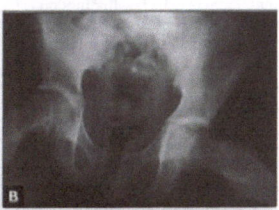

Figure 2. A, Klein's lines are drawn on the superior border of the femoral neck in this patient with slipped capital femoral epiphysis in the right hip. Note that the femoral head is below Kline's line on the affected right side, whereas a significant portion of the femoral head is above the line on the unaffected left side. B, Lateral radiograph of the right hip shows posterior displacement of the capital femoral epiphysis.

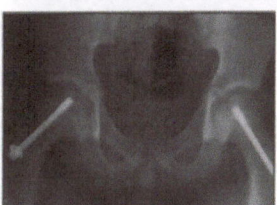

Figure 3. This patient with bilateral slipped capital femoral epiphysis has been treated using percutaneous in situ cannulated screw fixation.

Key references
1. Blanco D, Taylor B, Johnston CE: Comparison of single pin versus multiple pin fixation in treatment of slipped capital femoral epiphysis. J Pediatr Orthop 1992, 12:384.
2. Carney BT, Weinstein ST, Noble J: Long term follow-up of slipped capital femoral epiphysis. J Bone Joint Surg [Am] 1991, 73:667.
3. Jacobs B: Diagnosis and natural history of slipped capital femoral epiphysis. In Instructional Course Lectures vol 21. Rosemont, IL: American Academy of Orthopaedic Surgeons; 1972:167.
4. Loder RT, Richards BS, Shapiro PS, et al: Acute slipped capital femoral epiphysis: the importance of physeal stability. J Bone Joint Surg [Am] 1993, 75:1134.
5. Maurer R, Larsen I: Acute necrosis of cartilage in slipped capital femoral epiphysis. J Bone Joint Surg [Am] 1970, 52:39.
6. Meier MC, Meyer LC, Ferguson RL: Treatment of slipped capital femoral epiphysis with a spica cast. J Bone Joint Surg [Am] 1992, 74:1522.

R. Ward

Diagnosis

History

Most patients have a history of insidious onset and slow progression of back pain in the lumbar area. On clinical presentation, most patients have a long history of lumbar back pain with a more recent pain progression to the buttocks and lower extremities. Pain is exacerbated by standing, walking, and other activities with erect posture, and is relieved by lying supine or by lumbar flexion, *ie,* bending over while pushing a grocery cart. Patients may experience back, buttock, or leg pain and frequent numbness or "giving out" of the legs.

Physical Findings

The common findings—pain, numbness, and subjective weakness—during ambulation are referred to as *neurogenic claudication.* At physical examination, patients with stenosis may have neurologic findings (fewer than half of patients), pain with lumbar extension, and usually normal pulses. Tenderness may be elicited over the sciatic notches or sacroiliac regions. The lumbar spine range of motion and lordosis are usually reduced. Positive tension signs (straight leg raising) are infrequent; however, these may be positive if concurrent disk herniation or nerve root entrapment is present. Sensory and motor examination are usually normal in patients at rest, but postexercise examination may elicit subtle motor or sensory changes. Even in the presence of many symptoms, there may be few findings on physical examination. A thorough examination must be performed to rule out other conditions with referred pain to the lumbar spine and lower extremities.

Imaging and radiographic studies

Imaging studies confirm the clinical diagnosis. Plain radiographs are useful for detecting disk degeneration, disk space narrowing, loss of lordotic lumbar curvature, and facet abnormalities (*ie,* degeneration, subluxation). Advanced studies are more useful for preoperative planning. Computed tomography (CT), postmyelography CT, or magnetic resonance imaging (MRI) is needed to confirm neural element compression (Fig. 1). MRI is advantageous because it is noninvasive and is a very sensitive method to evaluate the soft tissue and bony elements contributing to the stenosis. Myelography is invasive and requires injection of contrast medium into the spinal canal; however, many spine surgeons consider myelography superior to plain CT or MRI for preoperative planning of lumbar decompression.

Complications

The natural history of mild cases is relatively stable; however, moderate to severe cases can progress and exhibit neurologic deficits, cauda equina syndrome, and possibly severe lower extremity weakness. Additionally, disabling pain may severely affect the patient's quality of life.

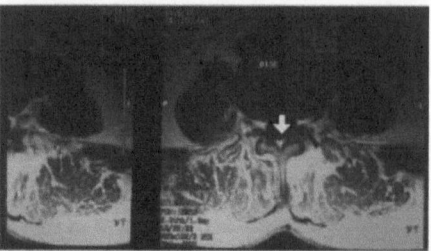

Figure 1. Axial magnetic resonance image of stenosis with hypertrophic facet (*arrow*).

Differential diagnosis

Pain in the back and lower extremities caused by lumbar spinal stenosis may be mimicked by vascular conditions (eg, peripheral vascular disease, aortic aneurysm); degenerative arthritis (hip or knee); spinal tumors (primary, metastatic, and epidural); Paget's disease; infection (vertebral, disk space, and epidural); diabetic neuropathy; cervical myelopathy; amyotrophic lateral sclerosis; peripheral compressive myelopathy; renal disorders; retroperitoneal tumors; and depression.

Etiology or pathophysiology

Lumbar spinal stenosis is usually caused by a reduction in the space available for the neural elements due to osseous or soft tissue filling the spinal canal. Two main types of stenosis are central stenosis (compression of the dural sac as a main component), and lateral stenosis (compression of the nerve root in the lateral recess, in the neural foramen, or lateral to the neural foramen). Narrowing of the spinal canal or neural foramina produces nerve root compression, nerve root ischemia, and progressive back and leg pain. Pathophysiology commonly begins with disk dehydration, which results in decreased disk height and bulging of the annulus fibrosus and ligamentum flavum into the spinal canal. Progressive degeneration leads to facet arthrosis with sclerosis and osteophyte overgrowth. The most common result is nerve root compression in the lateral recess when hypertrophic facet joints, ligamentum flavum, and a bulging annulus encroach on them. The degenerative process can be accompanied by the development of segmental instability. Central stenosis can be congenital (achondroplasia) or, more commonly, acquired (degenerative). It can also be posttraumatic, secondary to degenerative spondylolisthesis, or the result of other disease processes (eg, Paget's disease).

Epidemiology

The incidence of degenerative lumbar spinal stenosis ranges from approximately 2% to 8%. Symptoms usually develop in the fifth or sixth decades of life as a degenerative process. There is no gender predominance; however, lumbar spinal stenosis secondary to degenerative spondylolisthesis is four times more common in women.

Treatment

Nonsurgical

Nonsurgical treatment is directed at management of the patient's symptoms. The first line of treatment is nonsteroidal anti-inflammatory drugs (NSAIDs). At lower doses, NSAIDs reduce pain through an analgesic effect and at higher doses provide an anti-inflammatory effect on nerve root irritation. In patients with severe radicular symptoms, corticosteroids have been shown to have a potent anti-inflammatory effect; however, the benefits must be weighed against potential side effects such as osteonecrosis of the femoral head, hyperglycemia, and potential mental status changes in the elderly. Other medications used include muscle relaxants, antidepressants, and calcitonin. Physical therapy, such as a back-pain–relieving exercise program, aerobic exercises, or a combination of postural exercises in flexion with pelvic stabilization and aerobics is important. Weight loss and aerobic conditioning are highly beneficial in obese individuals. Patients with lumbar stenosis are well suited for an exercise bicycle. A brace or corset for immobilization can reduce back pain, particularly when associated with segmental instability or spondylolisthesis. Lumbar epidural steroids may be helpful for short-term relief but have not been shown to be effective in long-term studies.

Surgical

Surgical treatment is reserved primarily for patients in whom nonoperative treatment has failed. Preoperative planning requires an extensive review of the magnetic resonance image or postmyelographic computed tomography scan to determine the specific areas of neural element compression. Furthermore, a thorough work-up should identify any associated spondylolisthesis, segmental instability, or scoliosis that may require stabilization. Lumbar decompression surgery is primarily indicated in cases of progressive neurologic deficit, cauda equina syndrome, and disabling lower-extremity weakness. Surgical success rates as high as 85% have been reported but these rates may be reduced by inadequate decompression and stabilization. Surgical decompression involves undercutting the facet joints and pars interarticularis, with care taken to preserve at least 50% of the facet joints. A foraminotomy is usually necessary in patients with severe degenerative stenosis. Patients with associated spondylolisthesis or segmental instability (defined as more than 3 mm of motion between vertebrae on dynamic views) have been shown to benefit from arthrodesis with intertransverse autogenous bone grafting. Internal fixation is controversial and generally reserved for more physically active patients with higher degrees of instability. Postoperative complications may include infection, epidural hematoma, iatrogenic instability after wide decompression, and nonunion secondary to failure of grafting procedures.

Exercise and activity modification

Postural exercises in flexion with aerobic exercises are encouraged. Aerobic conditioning improves overall muscle tone and assists in weight loss. Patients with spinal stenosis are well suited for an exercise bicycle for pain relief by lumbar flexion.

Treatment aims

To relieve patient discomfort and to return patient to a tolerable quality of life. Surgical treatment is directed at reducing the compression of the neural elements and preventing progression of neurologic deficit and motor weakness.

Prognosis

The natural history of degenerative lumbar spinal stenosis has been demonstrated to be relatively stable in mild cases. In one study, the symptoms of approximately 70% of patients were unchanged at 4-year follow-up. Short-term studies have reported success rates as high as 85% in patients who required surgical decompression; however, data on long-term comparisons of nonoperative and operative interventions are needed.

Follow-up and management

All patients with lumbar spinal stenosis should be followed whether treated surgically or nonsurgically for potential progression of neurologic deficit. Patients treated nonsurgically may require prolonged NSAIDs in addition to continuous physical therapy, aerobic conditioning, and weight loss management. Surgically treated patients should be monitored for any postoperative complications as well as recurrent stenosis.

Key references

1. Hilibrand AS, Rand N: Degenerative lumbar stenosis: diagnosis and management. *J Am Acad Orthop Surg* 1999, 7:239–249.

2. Spivak JM: Degenerative lumbar stenosis. *J Bone Joint Surg* 1998, 80A:1053–1065.

3. Porter RW: Spinal stenosis and neurogenic claudication. *Spine* 1996, 21:2046–2052.

R. Ward

Diagnosis

History

Spondylolisthesis refers to the forward slippage of one vertebra on another. This condition is found most commonly at the lumbosacral junction. The average patient with spondylolisthesis presents in adulthood with a history of insidious onset of back pain with gradual progression of symptoms. Adults with spondylolisthesis may have a history of back pain, lower extremity weakness, and extremity pain and paresthesias (childhood spondylolisthesis is discussed in a separate section). While lower extremity complaints are common, objective neurologic deficits are found infrequently.

Physical findings

At the physical examination, patients may be found to have increased lumbar lordosis. There may be a palpable defect in the lower lumbar region (L4 or L5). Although neurologic deficits are uncommon, patients may exhibit a decrease in light touch sensation over the dorsum of the foot and weakness of the extensor hallucis longus correlating with L5 root irritation. This root is the most commonly involved and is seen with an L5-S1 spondylolisthesis. Tension signs (straight-leg raise) are usually negative on physical examination. Furthermore, patients rarely complain of loss of bowel or bladder function.

Imaging and laboratory studies

Initial investigation of patients with suspected spondylolisthesis consists of plain radiographs in the anteroposterior and lateral planes. Oblique radiographs may be useful to identify a defect in the pars interarticularis; however, the lateral radiograph will show approximately 80% of lesions. Based on radiographs, the severity of the slip in spondylolisthesis is based on the amount of slippage compared with the width of S1: **grade I**, 0% to 25%; **grade II**, 26% to 50%; **grade III**, 51% to 75%; **grade IV**, 76% to 100%; **grade V**, > 100% (spondyloptosis). Figure 1 is a radiograph of a patient with a grade I spondylolisthesis of L5 on S1. In patients with more occult slippage, computed tomography (CT) or single photon emission CT may be necessary to detect the spondylolysis. In patients with high-grade deformities, myelography, CT, and magnetic resonance imaging (MRI) may be used to determine the degree of compression on the neural elements.

Complications

Patients with high-grade slips may experience debilitating lumbar back pain and progressive neurologic deficits. In adults, the L5 nerve root is most commonly affected (because of an L5 on S1 slip). In severe cases, symptoms may progress to severe extremity pain with decreased sensation and weakness.

Differential diagnosis

Degenerative lumbar disk disease, spinal fracture, spinal tumor, herniated disk, spinal stenosis, spinal infection.

Etiology or pathophysiology

Spondylolysis is a defect in the pars interarticularis without displacement of a vertebra. Classification of spondylolisthesis and spondylolysis consists of five types: Type 1, dysplastic: a congenital abnormality of the upper sacrum or the arch of L5, permitting a slip to occur; Type 2, isthmic: lesions of the pars interarticularis (see below); Type 3, degenerative: a result of long-standing intersegmental instability; Type 4, traumatic: a result of fractures in area other than the pars interarticularis; Type 5, pathologic: a result of generalized or localized bone disease. The three lesions that cause Type 2 spondylolisthesis and spondylolysis are lytic—fatigue fracture of the pars interarticularis; elongated —pars interarticularis intact but elongated; and fracture—acute fracture of the pars). Isthmic spondylolisthesis, the most common type, results from spondylolysis of the pars interarticularis. It is seen more frequently at L5-S1. Development of the isthmic defect is considered to be due to a hereditary predisposition to fatigue or stress fracture of the pars. Isthmic spondylolisthesis is usually a developmental abnormality occuring in childhood; however, most patients do not seek evaluation until pain onset in adulthood. Increased incidence of spondylolisthesis and spondylolysis has been associated with sporting activities, including repetitive lumbar extension. Controversy exists as to the etiology of back pain in patients with spondylolisthesis. Suggested causes include segmental instability, disk degeneration at the level of the spondylolisthesis, and narrowing of the intervertebral foramen with nerve root compression.

Epidemiology

In a prospective study of 500 children, the incidence of spondylolysis was found to be 4.4%; this increased to 6% by young adulthood. Radiographically, 75% of the defects were evident by 6 years of age, and 74% of the patients with spondylolysis also demonstrated spondylolisthesis.

Treatment

Nonsurgical

Nonsurgical treatment consists primarily of rest, activity modification, lumbar corset, and back strengthening exercises. A back flexion exercise program is superior to extension exercise strengthening. Most patients with mild to moderate symptoms respond well to nonoperative treatment.

Surgical

Indications for surgical treatment include persistent severe back or leg pain. Although unusual, progressive deformity in the adult with worsening motor deficit and bowel or bladder dysfunction is also a surgical indication. In patients with severe, persistent lower back pain with or without radiculopathy who have not responded to nonoperative management, arthrodesis, may be indicated. A postero-lateral fusion with or without internal fixation is the most commonly performed procedure. Success rates of arthrodesis have been reported in excess of 90%.

Exercise and activity modification

Patients should be counseled on avoidance of aggravating activities, such as bending, stooping, and heavy lifting. A brief period of rest and immobilization with lumbar corset or brace may provide relief with acute severe pain. Back strengthening exercises should be continued daily. Aerobic conditioning is beneficial for both weight loss and overall strengthening.

Treatment aims
To provide symptomatic relief and prevent progressive neurologic deficit.

Prognosis
The success of nonsurgical treatment has been reported to be more than 60% in symptomatic patients. Success rates following arthrodesis are reported to be greater than 90%.

Follow-up and management
All patients with spondylolisthesis should be followed-up for evaluation of symptoms and for any progressive neurologic deficits.

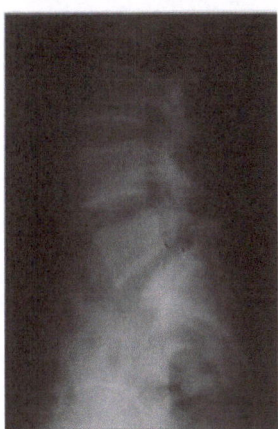

Figure 1. Radiograph of the lumbar spine shows a grade I spondylolisthesis with an anterior slip of approximately 25% of L5 on S1.

Key references
1. Frederickson BE, Baker D, McHolick WJ, et al.: The natural history of spondylolysis and spondylolisthesis. *J Bone Joint Surg* 1984, 66A:699–707.
2. Lauerman WC, Cain JE Jr: Isthmic spondylolisthesis in the adult. *J Am Acad Orthop Surg* 1996, 4:201–208.
3. Boxall D, Bradford DS, Winter RB, et al.: Management of severe spondylolisthesis in children and adolescents. *J Bone Joint Surg* 1979, 61A:479.

Diagnosis

History

Children with spondylolisthesis generally have a history of repetitive episodes of low back pain. Patients may have experienced postural deformity and abnormal gait previously. A history of trauma is common, and patients often seek treatment after an episode of low back pain after a minor trauma; however, history of severe trauma is unusual. The onset of symptoms often coincides closely with the adolescent growth spurt (10 to 15 years of age).

Physical findings

Children with low back pain and spondylolisthesis may experience hamstring tightness, spinal deformity, and an abnormal, peculiar, gait pattern because of tight hamstrings. Patients frequently are participants in sports that involve repetitive forced lumbar extension (*ie*, gymnastics). On examination, patients may exhibit profound hamstring tightness with a pelvic waddling gait. Radicular findings may be present, particularly of the L5 nerve root and the cauda equina. Patients often exhibit a hyperlordosis of the upper spine with a kyphosis of the lumbosacral junction. A classic finding of "heart-shaped" buttocks is occasionally present.

Imaging and laboratory studies

Radiographs in the anteroposterior and especially the lateral planes are usually adequate. Oblique radiographs of the lumbar spine may be necessary to view the possible defect in the pars interarticularis. The commonly used "Scotty dog" sign of LaChapelle as seen on the oblique appears as a defect in the collar around the dog's neck (pars interarticularis). The slip in spondylolisthesis is based on the degree of anterior translation of one vertebra on another: **grade I,** 0% to 25%; **grade II,** 26% to 50%; **grade III,** 51% to 75%; **grade IV,** 76% to 100%; **grade V,** > 100%. Grade V is also referred to as *spondyloptosis*. Children with a dome-shaped vertebral sacrum and trapezoidal L5 vertebral body have a greater tendency for further slip and continued symptoms. Standing flexion and extension views of the lumbosacral junction may demonstrate the presence of instability and excessive motion. Radiographs may reveal a defect in the pars interarticularis with elongation of the pars (Type 1—dysplastic) or as a disruption of the pars (Type 2—isthmic). In late adolescence, disk space narrowing and sclerosis of the anterior lip of the sacrum may be present. Spondylolysis that is suspected clinically but cannot be detected radiographically may be detected with bone scans. Bone scans can help to detect the acute fracture and to distinguish between patients with an established nonunion from those who are in the healing process.

Complications

Although most slips are stable, some patients may have continued slippage with progressive lumbar deformity, gait abnormalities, and possible neurologic impairments. In patients with the dysplastic (Type 1) spondylolisthesis, further slippage is much more likely to occur. Additional slippage in as many as 50% of patients has been reported.

Differential diagnosis

Spina bifida occulta; thoracic kyphosis; Scheuermann's disease.

Etiology or pathophysiology

Two types of spondylolisthesis are described in children. Type 1 is dysplastic; Type 2 is isthmic. The dysplastic type is the result of congenital defects at the lumbosacral joint, and the isthmic type is a fatigue fracture with a suspected hereditary component. An episode of trauma often initiates the onset of symptoms; however, there seldom is a history of severe injury. It has been suggested that sheer stresses are greater on the pars interarticularis when the lumbar spine is extended. Patients involved in sports with repetitive lumbar extension are at increased risk for spondylolysis.

Epidemiology

The incidence of spondylolysis has been found to be 4.4% in 6-year-olds, increasing to 6% at young adulthood. Despite an average incidence of 5% in the general population, a pars interarticularis defect is rare in an infant.

Treatment

Nonsurgical

Patients with low-grade slips (< 50%) usually respond to nonoperative treatment that consists primarily of activity modification and exercises. Patients with grade I slips usually can return to sports; however, patients with grade II slips are generally restricted from contact sports. Occasionally, patients with low-grade slips may require surgery because of intractable pain despite conservative treatment.

Surgical

Surgical treatment is reserved for patients with low-grade slips who have intractable pain and have failed conservative treatment. Prophylactic fusion is recommended in children with a slippage of > 50% (grades III, IV, and V). This often necessitates posterolateral fusion in situ from L4 to S1 without instrumentation. Reduction of spondylolisthesis is discouraged because of reported 20% to 30% incidence of L5 nerve root injuries postreduction.

Exercise and activity modification

Patients with grade I and grade II slips are allowed to return to exercise and sporting activities. Patients with grade II slips are generally restricted from contact sports. Higher-grade slips usually require restriction from exercise and sports, and surgery is recommended.

Treatment aims

To alleviate discomfort and to prevent progressive slippage with resultant progressive neurologic dysfunction and gait and postural abnormalities.

Prognosis

Females are at greater risk for additional slippage than are males. Progression occurs primarily during the adolescent growth spurt (10 to 15 years of age). Reports of patients treated nonoperatively reveal > 80% success (patients with no pain on long-term follow-up). Success rates of posterolateral fusion have been reported between 90% and 100%. At 18-year follow-up of patients with high-grade slips (grades III, IV) treated nonoperatively, 45% of patients avoid heavy lifting; job choices of 36% have been influenced by it; and many limit their recreational activities.

Follow-up and management

All patients with spondylolysis and spondylolisthesis should be followed for progressive pain and deformity. Adolescents represent less than 10% of cases requiring stabilization surgery; however, patients with Type I dysplastic spondylolisthesis should be followed closely because further slippage is much more likely in this type.

Key references

1. Boxall D, Bradford DS, Winter RB, et al: Management of severe spondylolisthesis in children and adolescents. *J Bone Joint Surg* 1979, 61A:479–486.
2. Hensinger RN, Lang JR, MacEwen GD: Surgical management of spondylolisthesis in children and adolescents. *Spine* 1976, 1:207–215.
3. Hensinger RN: Spondylolysis and spondylolisthesis in children and adolescents. *J Bone Joint Surg* 1989, 71A:1098–1115.
3. Saraste H: Long-term clinical and radiological follow-up of spondylolysis and spondylolisthesis. *J Pediatr Orthop* 1987, 7:631–640.
4. Lauerman WC, Cain JE: Isthmic spondylolisthesis in the adult. *J Am Acad Orthop Surg* 1996, 4:210–208.

Diagnosis

History
Fall on an outstretched arm.

Localized elbow pain.

Physical findings
Nondisplaced and mild fractures have tenderness to the medial and lateral columns of the supracondylar humerus. Diffuse swelling and joint effusion may be present. Displaced fractures demonstrate obvious deformity. Neurologic compromise may be present. If distal pulses are absent, it is important to note whether the hand remains warm and pink because of collateral circulation.

Imaging and laboratory studies
Radiographs: An anteroposterior radiograph with the elbow extended and a lateral radiograph of the elbow flexed to 90° are standard. If obvious deformity is present, do not attempt to flex and extend the elbow. A line extending down from the anterior humeral shaft should bisect the ossific nucleus of the capitellum. Visualization of the posterior fat pad indicates a joint effusion, which is common with occult or nondisplaced fractures. Radiographs of the remainder of the forearm and arm may be needed if the presence of other injuries cannot be clinically determined.

Complications
Compartment syndrome.

Median, radial, ulna, and anterior interosseous nerve injuries.

Brachial artery injury.

Growth disturbance of the distal humerus or avascular necrosis of the distal fragment (unusual).

Cubitus varus often resulting from malunion.

Elbow stiffness.

Differential diagnosis
Transcondylar (physeal) fractures.
Elbow dislocation.
T-condylar fracture.

Etiology or pathophysiology
Extension-type supracondylar humerus fractures (Fig. I) are usually secondary to a fall on an outstretched arm. Flexion type injuries occur secondary to a fall directly on the posterior elbow area. These are relatively rare.

Epidemiology
Supracondylar fractures encompass about 80% of elbow fractures in children. Peak incidence occurs in boys ages 5 to 10 years.
Extension fractures are classified as Type I (minimally displaced), Type II (displaced with intact posterior cortex), and Type III (minimal or no contact between the fragments).

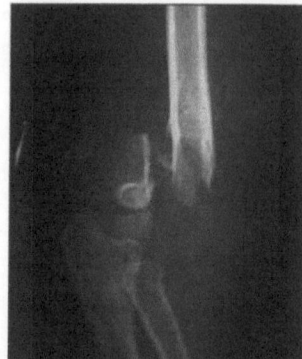

Figure I. Supracondylar fracture of the humerus.

Treatment

Nonsurgical

Type I extension injuries can be treated in a long arm cast with the elbow flexed to 90°. The carrying angle should be assessed before immobilization. Immobilization lasting 3 weeks is sufficient.

Surgical

Type II extension injuries must be reduced if there is loss of normal carrying angle or the capitellum is posterior to the anterior humeral line. General anesthesia and image intensification are required. Full flexion usually reduces the fracture. The carrying angle should be checked after reduction. To maintain reduction, the elbow must be immobilized in at least 120° of flexion or percutaneously pinned and splinted. Fixation allows for immobilization of the elbow in greater extension; this is important if there is any question about further swelling affecting the neurovascular status.

Type III extension injuries (Fig. 2A) must be operatively reduced and pinned. If an adequate closed reduction cannot achieved, open reduction is necessary. This is common for displaced flexion type injuries. Exploration of the brachial artery is necessary for absent distal pulses and signs of ischemia. If pulses are absent but the hand is pink and warm with full active motion of the digits, exploration is probably not necessary. The carrying angle should always be checked. Pin fixation can consist of two crossed pins (medial and lateral) (Fig. 2B,C) or of three lateral pins if there is concern about safely placing the medial pin near the ulna nerve. Olecranon pin traction is considered for severe soft tissue injury or markedly comminuted fractures.

Treatment aims
To maintain both full function and a normal carrying angle.

Prognosis
Although cosmetic and functional results are usually excellent, mild residual stiffness may occur.

Follow-up and management
If the surgery is uneventful and the fracture uncomplicated, the first office visit takes place 3 weeks after surgery, at which time the pins are removed. Usually a sling or removable splint is placed for early range of motion. If range of motion does not significantly improve after 2 to 3 weeks, formal physical therapy is considered.

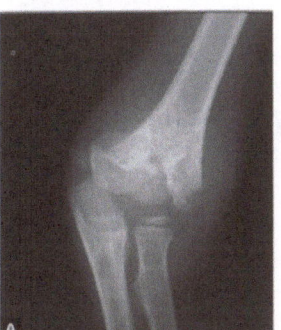
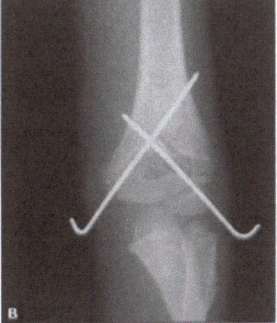
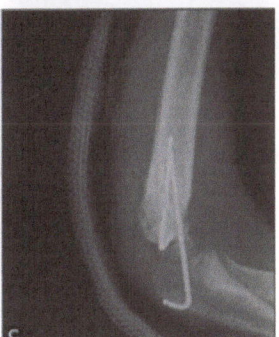

Figure 2. A, Type III extension supracondylar humerus fracture. Postoperative radiograph with the elbow taken after closed reduction and percutaneous pinning. B, antero-posterior (AP) and C, lateral views.

Key references
1. Wilkins KE: Supracondylar fractures of the distal humerus. In *Fractures in Children.* Edited by Rockwood CA, Wilkins KE, Beaty JH. Philadelphia: Lippincott–Raven; 1996:669–752.

Diagnosis

History

A tarsal coalition is a congenital bony, cartilaginous, or fibrous linkage between two tarsal bones (calcaneous, cuboid, navicular, talus). Patients present clinically with vague aching that is localized to the subtalar joint. Activity worsens the pain, and rest reduces it.

Physical findings

The symptomatic foot with tarsal coalition has been called peroneal spastic flatfoot because the foot is everted, the peroneal muscles are shortened, and passive inversion of the foot causes pain. The term is inaccurate because the peroneal muscles are not in true spasm. Subtalar motion may be limited, especially with talocalcaneal coalitions. Pes planus may be present.

Imaging and laboratory studies

The initial radiographs should include anteroposterior, lateral, and oblique views of the foot. In calcaneonavicular coalitions, the oblique radiograph best shows osseous bars; most cartilaginous coalitions can be identified by the narrowing present between the navicular and the calcaneus. This coalition can also be seen on the lateral view as elongation of the superior anterior calcaneus to the middle of the navicular, the so-called "anteater's nose" sign. Talocalcaneal coalitions are more difficult to see on plain radiographs. On the lateral view, the middle facet of the subtalar joint may be absent, but this may be a normal finding because of facet obliquity. Secondary signs, such as talar beaking, concavity of the inferior neck of the talus, and narrowing of the subtalar joint, suggest subtalar coalition. Further imaging studies should be obtained. Computed tomography in the coronal plane is extremely helpful in the visualization of subtalar coalitions and can complement plain radiographs to detect multiple coalitions. When radiographs and computed tomography scans are negative in the face of a clinical coalition, magnetic resonance imaging can be considered to detect fibrous coalitions.

Complications

In untreated talocalcaneal coalitions, a ball-and-socket ankle may develop to compensate for the loss of subtalar motion. Surgically treated coalitions may be complicated by recurrence.

Differential diagnosis

Subtalar osteochondral fracture.
Early degenerative joint disease.
Juvenile rheumatoid arthritis.
Osteomyelitis of the tarsus.
Septic arthritis of the subtalar joint.

Etiology

The cause of tarsal coalition is failure of differentiation and segmentation of the primitive mesenchyme of the tarsus during embryologic development. The reason for this congenital failure is unknown. The onset of symptoms seems related to the age at which the coalition begins to ossify; this suggests that symptoms are related to decreased joint motion.

Epidemiology

The incidence of tarsal coalition is estimated at 1% to 2.9%. The most common coalitions are the calcaneonavicular and talocalcaneal. Other coalitions are extremely rare. The calcaneonavicular coalition (Fig. 1) becomes symptomatic from age 8 to 12 years and is bilateral in 60% of cases. The talocalcaneal coalition (Fig. 2) becomes symptomatic between 12 and 16 years and is bilateral in 50% of cases. Inheritance is thought to be autosomal dominant, with close to full penetrance.

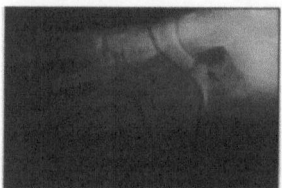

Figure 1. Calcaneonavicular osseous tarsal coalition.

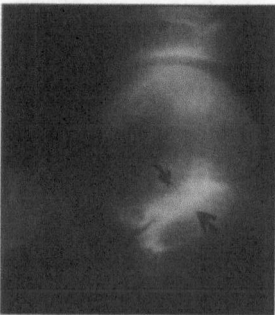

Figure 2. Talocalcaneal tarsal coalition obliterating most of the subtalar joint.

180

Treatment

Nonsurgical

Conservative measures for pain relief are the initial treatment for tarsal coalition. This includes arch supports, plastizote shoe inserts, and reduction in activities that produce symptoms. Patients who do not respond may be placed in a short-leg walking cast for a trial of 3 to 6 weeks for pain control. Casting trials may be repeated for patients whose symptoms recur. About one third of patients can be managed by conservative measures alone.

Surgical

Patients with persistent symptoms in whom conservative measures fail may be considered for surgical treatment. If there are no degenerative changes, talonavicular coalitions undergo block resection with interposition of the extensor digitorum brevis into the defect. After surgery, the foot is immobilized in a cast for 2 weeks; weight bearing begins 4 weeks after surgery. This procedure is successful in 80% of patients, and the best results are seen in those with cartilaginous coalitions who are younger than 16 years of age at time of surgery. The surgical treatment of talocalcaneal coalition is more controversial. If no degenerative changes are present and computed tomography confirms that the coalition involves less than 50% of the articular surface of the subtalar joint, then the coalition can be resected with interposition of a fat graft. Results are good for 70% of patients, but long-term follow-up is lacking. Patients who have intractable pain with degenerative changes associated with a valgus heel may benefit from a calcaneal osteotomy, but triple arthrodesis is indicated in patients with symptomatic degenerative disease who have reached late adolescence.

Treatment aims
To relieve the pain of tarsal coalition.

Prognosis
The prognosis is favorable for patients treated surgically before degenerative changes are apparent.

Follow-up and management
The patient is followed monthly for three visits after surgery and can usually return to normal activities within 2 months of surgery. Radiographs are taken 6 months after surgery to detect recurrence of the coalition. Yearly follow-up is needed until the patient reaches skeletal maturity.

Key references

1. Harris RI, Beath T: Etiology of peroneal spastic flat foot. J Bone Joint Surg [Br] 1948, 30:624.
2. Horn DB, Pizzutillo PD, Wechsler RJ, et al.: Magnetic resonance imaging in the diagnosis of tarsal coalition. Proceedings of the American Orthopedic Association, Sun Valley, Idaho, 1994.
3. Jayakumar S, Cowell HR: Rigid flatfoot. Clin Orthop 1977, 122:77.
4. Leonard MA: The inheritance of tarsal coalition and its relationship to spastic flat foot. J Bone Joint Surg [Br] 1974, 56:520.
5. McCormack T, Olney B, Asher M: Long-term follow-up of middle facet talocalcaneal coalition resections. In Proceedings of the Pediatric Orthopaedic Society of North America. Memphis, TN: Pediatric Orthopaedic Society of North America; 1994.
6. Oestreich AE, Mize WA, Crawford AH, et al.: The "anteater nose": direct sign of calcaneonavicular coalition on the lateral radiograph. J Pediatr Orthop 1987, 7:709.
7. Stormont DM, Peterson HA: The relative incidence of tarsal coalition. Clin Orthop 1983, 181:28.

Diagnosis

History

Most patients with thoracolumbar fractures have been involved in high-energy injuries, such as motor vehicle collisions or falls from significant heights. They often have associated injuries, both abdominal and orthopedic. Elderly patients can sustain compression fractures from trivial trauma due to severe osteoporosis.

Physical findings

Patients may or may not present with varying degrees of paralysis. The presence of pain depends on the type, level, and severity of injury. A thorough physical examination that includes a complete neurologic assessment is indicated. Reflexes to test include the superficial abdominal reflexes (T7 to T10, above the umbilicus; T11 to L1 below the umbilicus), cremasteric (T12 to L1), knee jerk (L3 and L4), ankle jerk (S1), anal wink (S2 to S4), bulbocavernosus (S3 and S4), and plantar response (Babinski, brain-cord continuity).

The back must be palpated, and step-off or tenderness to palpation should be assessed. Rectal tone must be documented. In cases of suspected spinal shock, bulbocavernosus reflex should be checked and properly documented. The absence of the reflex indicates spinal shock. The return of the reflex signifies the end of spinal shock. The surgeon should check for associated injuries, such as calcaneus fractures in falls or abdominal injuries in motor vehicle accidents. An abdominal contusion is a diagnostic clue for a spine fracture, specifically the flexion-distraction (lap belt) type of injury.

A complete trauma work-up is indicated in these patients; the basics must be adhered to. Vital signs indicating neurogenic shock must be addressed. This state of relative hypotension results from a loss of sympathetic tone with unopposed vagal parasympathetic vasodilatation. Its hallmark is bradycardia despite hypotension. If tachycardia is present, another source for the hypotension should be sought.

Imaging and laboratory studies

Standard anteroposterior and lateral radiographs of the thorax or lumbar area should be obtained (Fig. 1). Widening of the interpedicular distance on an anteroposterior view is a subtle finding, indicating a fracture of the vertebral body. The lateral radiograph is used to assess the loss of vertebral height and kyphosis. Retropulsion of bony fragments can also be assessed with radiography, although computed tomography (CT) is best. The CT scan must include sagittal and coronal reconstructions. Magnetic resonance imaging is of occasional benefit in the patient whose plain films are normal but who have severe back pain or a neurologic deficit attributable to the accident.

Complications

Failure to diagnose a thoracolumbar fracture could result in a neurologic injury, progressive deformity, and chronic pain. Complications are mainly neurologic. Surgical treatment has risks associated with the surgery and hardware, such as failure of fixation, neurologic deficit, infection, nonunion, and flat back syndrome.

Differential diagnosis

The diagnosis is usually straightforward, and the complexity in diagnosis lies in the prompt recognition of the injury in a trauma patient. Other injuries that can give a picture of neurologic injury are injuries to the brain itself or peripheral nerve injuries. Paralysis of a limb may be due to fractures in the limb itself or injury to the nerve. The patient must be evaluated for all of these injuries.

Etiology or pathophysiology

Flexion-rotation, shear, flexion-distraction and extension type injuries. The spine has been considered a three-column entity, as described by Denis, and is divided into the posterior, middle, and anterior columns. The posterior column features all the posterior bony elements and ligaments to include the ligamentum flavum. The middle column consists of the posterior third of the body/annulus and posterior longitudinal ligament. The anterior column comprises two thirds of the body/annulus and the anterior longitudinal ligament. The compression fracture involves only the anterior column. Stable burst fractures are compression fractures that involve the anterior and middle columns. An unstable burst fracture is a compression fracture involving all three columns. The Chance fracture is a flexion-distraction type of injury. Neurologic injury can also be classified according to root or cord involvement. Cord injury is then classified as complete or incomplete. In complete cord syndromes are anterior cord syndrome, posterior cord syndrome, central cord syndrome, and Brown-Sequard syndrome.

Epidemiology

More than 1 million spine injuries occur annually in the United States. The group most commonly affected is male patients 15 to 35 years of age. Spine fractures account for 50,000 of the 1 million injuries. Only 20% of these spine fractures have neurologic deficits. The thoracolumbar area is the most common site of vertebral column injuries. Compression fractures account for about 50% of spine fractures in any given series. Noncontiguous spine fractures are present 20% of the time. In 10% to 50% of cases, fracture of the skull or long bones has also occurred. An associated cardiopulmonary injury has an incidence of 40%.

Treatment

Nonsurgical

Nonsurgical treatment of thoracolumbar fractures is restricted to injuries considered stable. These injuries must not have the potential for progressive deformity or neurologic injury when the patient ambulates with external immobilization. The usual immobilization device is a hyperextension thoracolumbosacral orthosis for approximately 3 months. Occasionally, the thigh must be incorporated into the brace for lower lumbar injuries that can be treated with bracing.

Surgical

All patients exhibiting neurologic injury who present within 8 hours of injury should receive steroids according to the National Acute Spinal Cord Injury Study protocol by Bracken. This entails giving the patient a corticosteroid bolus of 30 mg/kg of body weight, followed by an infusion of 5.4 mg/k/h for 23 hours. Efficacy of corticosteroid treatment has been shown only for blunt cord injury. It is not indicated for pure root injuries.

The decision to operate on a thoracolumbar fracture is based on certain factors. As a general rule, unstable fractures with or without a neurologic deficit, whether complete or incomplete, should be treated surgically to stabilize the spine. The difficulty arises in determining the exact stability of certain fracture patterns. For compression fractures, many authors have stated that if there is greater than 40% to 50% loss of height or greater than 30° of kyphosis, the spine should be stabilized and the deformity corrected. This can be accomplished by a posterior approach with distraction instrumentation. Burst fractures associated with greater than 50% canal compromise, greater than 30° of kyphosis, or greater than 40% to 50% loss of height should also be stabilized.

Surgical stabilization is performed through a posterior approach, an anterior approach, or a combined approach; all approaches use instrumentation with fusion of the involved levels. The posterior approach is considered the indirect reduction method, although this can be combined with posterolateral decompression. The direct approach for reduction and decompression is through the anterior approach, which uses a retroperitoneal dissection. If surgery is delayed because of other factors, the indirect method will often be unsuccessful in decompressing the spinal canal. In these "late" surgeries, the anterior approach is more useful.

Exercise and activity modification

The patient is usually restricted from exercise until the fracture has healed (usually 12 to 16 weeks). Life-long activity modifications may be needed, depending on the type of injury and treatment. Fusion is a part of surgical intervention. Fusion can result in loss of some motion depending on the level and number of vertebral bodies fused, which directly influences the patient's ability to participate in certain activities.

Treatment aims

To restore alignment and stability of the spine and to restore and protect neurologic function are the main foci of treatment.

Prognosis

Varies with type and severity of injury. The main prognostic factor is whether a neurologic deficit is present and whether it is complete or incomplete. The steroid protocol has been shown to improve the neurologic outcome of patients with cord injuries. Approximately 75% of patients with central cord syndromes have functional motor recovery; only 10% with an anterior cord injury have any functional recovery. The Brown-Sequard syndrome is associated with the best prognosis; more than 90% of patients have some functional motor recovery.

Follow-up and management

All patients need long-term follow-up, which should include social worker and physical medicine and rehabilitation physician. Surgical patients require bracing after surgery for approximately 12 weeks. Muscle tone and joint mobility should be maintained as best as possible, especially in paraplegic patients. Self-catheterization should be taught to patients with bladder dysfunction. Once the fracture has healed and the patient no longer needs a brace, physical therapy should be initiated in capable patients.

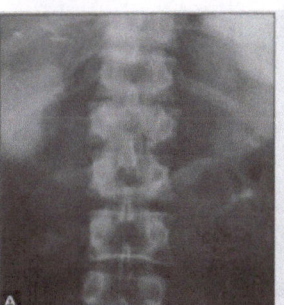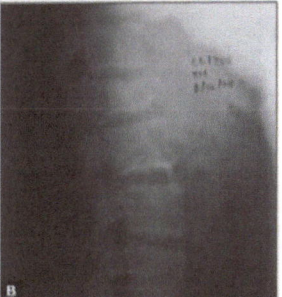

Figure 1. A, Anteroposterior (AP) and B, lateral views of an L1 burst fracture.

Key references

1. Spivak JM, Vaccaro AR, Cotler JM: Thoracolumbar spine trauma, I: evaluation and classification. J Am Acad Orthop Surg 1995, 3:345–352.

2. Spivak JM, Vaccaro AR, Cotler JM: Thoracolumbar spine trauma, II: principles of management. J Am Acad Orthop Surg 1995, 3:353–360.

Diagnosis

History

The force involved in causing a tibial shaft fracture can be applied directly or indirectly to the shin. Direct forces against the shin are more often high energy, as seen in an increasing number of motor vehicle crashes and pedestrian injuries. These injuries are usually open fractures that involve various degrees of soft tissue damage. Lower-energy shaft fractures are usually closed injuries that are associated with lesser soft tissue damage and result from short-distance falls or recreational activities. With fracture of both the tibia and fibula, the patient usually feels pain when the fractures occur and sees the leg deformed by the injury. When the patient attempts to walk after the event, placing weight on the injured extremity, severe pain is common.

Physical findings

Most tibial shaft fractures present as a deformity of the leg, especially if the fibula is also broken. The most common deformity pattern in a closed fracture is shortening, valgus angulation at the fracture, and external rotation of the distal fragment. Because of the subcutaneous position of the medial surface of the tibia, swelling, bruising, and ecchymosis are often present soon after injury. Direct nerve and vessel injury are uncommon after a closed shaft fracture. Nevertheless, a thorough baseline neurovascular examination of the extremity should be performed before any treatment is instituted. Results of subsequent evaluations can then be compared with those of the baseline examination to allow early detection of a compartment syndrome of the leg. The index of suspicion for nerve or vessel injury should be high during assessment of an open shaft fracture. The more severe the soft tissue injury, the greater the likelihood of direct nerve or vessel damage.

Imaging and laboratory studies

Simple orthogonal radiographs of the leg are usually all that is required to establish the presence of a shaft fracture (Fig. 1). Internal and external oblique radiographs may also be obtained to define the true fracture deformity and configuration. Computed tomography and magnetic resonance imaging should rarely be used to evaluate a tibial shaft fracture. When there is concern that a vascular injury has occurred with the fracture, a careful examination of both the dorsalis pedis and posterior tibial pulses can be supplemented with Doppler and, rarely, arteriographic studies. A device to measure intracompartmental pressure should be available for the evaluation of shaft fractures with significant soft tissue injury. These fractures have a higher risk for developing a compartment syndrome. Finally, a picture of the injured leg, especially if the injury is open, can facilitate the planning of treatment without the need to repeatedly examine the open wound after it has been dressed and splinted.

Complications

Complications are generally related to the extent of the presenting soft tissue and bone injury or to the treatment selected for the combined injuries. A simple closed fracture of the shaft without neurovascular injury can still be accompanied by such healing problems as malunion, delayed union, and nonunion. Open fractures present the additional challenge of wound contamination, which must be urgently addressed so that acute and chronic infection of the bone and soft tissue is prevented. Such infection could lead to an infected but united fracture, an infected nonunion, or amputation. After a shaft fracture, injured muscle can swell, leading to an increase in compartment pressure in any of the four compartments of the leg. If the pressure increases substantially, muscle ischemia may occur, resulting in muscle death and fibrosis. Such phenomena may cause muscle weakness, limited joint motion, or fibrous ankylosis.

Differential diagnosis

It is uncommon to mistake a tibial shaft fracture in the midportion of the leg for any other injury, especially if a deformity is present. More proximal and distal skeletal injuries must be differentiated from injuries that involve the knee or ankle joint. It should be assumed that puncture wounds on the medial border of the shin and extensive abrasions of the leg communicate with an open tibial shaft fracture until radiographs disprove the assumption.

Etiology or pathophysiology

A bimodal energy pattern is involved in the creation of a tibial shaft fracture. Low-energy injuries usually cause a fracture by means of torsional forces indirectly applied to the leg. Fracture patterns tend to be simpler, and soft tissue injury is mild to moderate. High-energy fractures more often result from direct trauma to the shin. Bone and soft tissue injuries tend to be severe and often are associated with wound contamination.

Epidemiology

The tibia is the most commonly fractured long bone of the body. Because of this frequency, myriad forms of treatment have been devised to achieve osseous healing with minimal complications. Many an orthopedist has been humbled attempting to achieve union in a "simple tibial shaft fracture."

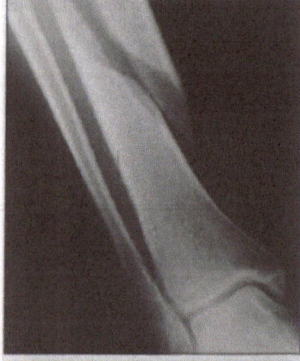

Figure 1. Radiograph of a tibial shaft fracture.

Treatment

Nonsurgical

Most tibial shaft fractures are still treated nonsurgically. Most low-energy closed fractures can be treated successfully with a closed reduction and casting. Weight bearing on the casted leg can begin when the pain allows. Early exchange of the cast for a weight-bearing orthosis is common. When the stability of the fracture reduction is problematic, weight bearing can be delayed until fracture stability has increased with callus formation. Higher-energy closed fractures and open fractures may be less amenable to nonsurgical treatment because of the extent of fracture instability caused by soft tissue injury. If nonsurgical treatment is initially undertaken in these situations, close follow-up of the patient is important in order to detect early loss of fracture reduction.

Surgical

An enormous amount of trauma literature exists on the operative treatment of tibial shaft fractures. Both simple and complex forms of external fixation have been applied to this injury, especially when the fracture has been open. An interlocking intramedullary nail has gained popularity in the treatment of closed and less severe open fractures of the tibial shaft. The number of proponents of cerclage and plate fixation of acute fractures has decreased as the results of nail and nonoperative treatment have become known. Open fractures of the shaft still require thorough cleansing and antibiotics to prevent osseous infection.

Exercise and activity modification

The initiation of early weight bearing in the treatment of tibial shaft fractures was one of the major advances in the care of this common injury. Improving muscle blood flow and function during fracture treatment by weight bearing was found to stimulate tibial healing. Tobacco use and poorly controlled diabetes are known to retard normal fracture healing in the tibial shaft.

Treatment aims

Closed tibial fracture: to restore normal function without pain within a reasonable period after injury. Open tibial fracture: to prevent infection. If bone and soft tissue infection can be prevented, then normal function after injury may be achieved if the zone of soft and hard tissue injury is not great. With good fracture care, the primary determinant of postinjury function should be the degree of injury.

Prognosis

The average time to clinical and radiographic union in a closed fracture is 16 weeks. Healing times in open shaft fractures vary depending on the extent of injury. Severe open injuries that are complicated by infection may lead to transtibial amputation if the infection cannot be controlled or eradicated.

Follow-up and management

Close follow-up soon after injury is important in treating both open and closed tibial shaft fractures. Closed fractures that are treated nonoperatively must be assessed to determine that the closed treatment maintains a satisfactory fracture reduction. Closed or open fractures that are treated operatively must be evaluated for fracture reduction and infection. Early rather than late interventions to address fracture malreduction or infection invariably lead to better long-term results.

Key references

1. Behrens F, Searls K: External fixation of the tibia. *J Bone Joint Surg* 1986, 68B:246–254.
2. Nicoll EA: Fractures of the tibial shaft. *J Bone Joint Surg* 1964, 46B:373–387.
3. Sarmiento A, Gersten LM, Sobol PA, et al.: Tibial shaft fractures treated with functional braces: experience with 780 fractures. *J Bone Joint Surg* 1989, 71B:602–609.

Diagnosis

History
The infant with torticollis presents with a nonpainful, fixed rotation of the neck caused by contracture of the sternocleidomastoid muscle. Presentation is usually between birth and age 3 weeks. Active rotation of the head to the side of the contracture is limited. The child prefers to sleep in the prone position to accommodate the fixed head position.

Physical findings
The contracted sternocleidomastoid muscle is shortened, thereby pulling the head toward the shoulder and rotating the chin away to the opposite side. Early in presentation, a nontender fusiform swelling is often contained in the distal end of the muscle; this gradually enlarges over several weeks and resolves in approximately 6 months (Fig. 1). Untreated patients will gradually develop flattening of the ipsilateral face and the contralateral occiput from external pressure of sleeping surfaces.

Imaging and laboratory studies
An anteroposterior and lateral radiograph of the cervical spine will be normal in patients with congenital muscular torticollis but should be taken to rule out congenital anomalies of the cervical spine, which can also cause torticollis.

Complications
If the neck contracture remains untreated, the asymmetry of the face worsens as the skeleton grows. The face on the affected side is relatively shortened, the eyes and ears are at different levels, and a cervical-thoracic scoliosis concave toward the side of the contracture may develop.

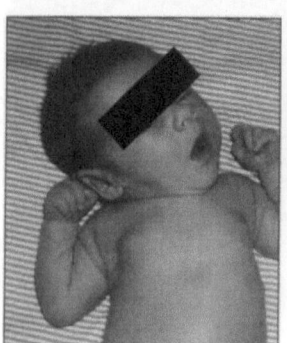

Figure 1. Torticollis in a newborn male infant. There is fusiform muscle swelling at the base of the right sternocleido-mastoid muscle. The head is in the "cocked-robin" position, with the face turned to the left and the head tilted to the right. This patient was treated with gentle stretching exercises of the neck performed by the parents.

Differential diagnosis
Postural torticollis.
Cervicothoracic hemivertebrae.
Unilateral atlantooccipital fusion.
Unilateral absence of C-1.
Klippel-Fiel syndrome.
Cervical fracture.
Rotatory subluxation of C-1 on C-2.
Spontaneous hyperemic subluxation of C-1 (Grisel's syndrome).
Rheumatoid arthritis.
Acute calcification of cervical disk.
Cervical lymphadenitis.
Syringomyelia.
Cervical spinal cord or posterior fossa tumors.

Etiology
Intramuscular fibrosis causes the clinical shortening and contracture of sternocleidomastoid muscle, but the cause of the fibrosis is controversial. Similar fibrosis can be induced in animals by venous occlusion of a muscle. The most current theory is that the sternocleidomastoid muscle in congenital muscular torticollis has undergone a compartment syndrome in utero.

Epidemiology
Torticollis is rare, and a family history of torticollis is infrequent. It is more common in girls than in boys. The right side of the neck is involved approximately 75% of the time. Breech position and difficult forceps delivery seem to be risk factors for congenital muscular torticollis. Associated developmental dislocation of the hip may be seen in 20% of cases.

Treatment

Nonsurgical

Passive stretching of the contracted muscle is begun by the parents after instruction from physical therapists. With the neck in a comfortably hyperextended position, the infant's head is gently pushed toward the shoulder opposite the contracted muscle, and the head is rotated toward the shoulder on the side of the contracted muscle. The exercises are done four times a day, with 15 repetitions for each exercise, and the infant's neck is held in maximum stretch for each exercise for 10 seconds. The infant's crib should be positioned so that the child must look toward the affected position for toys or mobiles. The prone sleeping position is to be avoided.

Surgical

When the torticollis does not respond to stretching exercises, surgical release of the sternocleidomastoid muscle is indicated. Release of the proximal pole of the muscle is more cosmetic than a complete distal release but is technically more difficult. The "V" contour of the neck can be preserved with a distal release if there is complete section of the clavicular insertion but only lengthening of the sternal portion. The correction is held with a cast or a brace, and exercises are continued after immobilization to prevent recurrence.

Treatment aims
To rule out osseous causes and other secondary causes of torticollis.
To treat muscular torticollis as early as possible with stretching exercises.
To restore full active range of motion to the neck of the infant.

Prognosis
If exercises are begun in the first year of life and parental compliance is good, then an average of 80% of patients will show correction of their torticollis. If treatment is delayed until the patient is older than 1 year, if facial asymmetry is present, and if greater than 30° of neck motion is lost, surgery is necessary because it is unlikely that exercise could correct the torticollis.

Follow-up and management
Regular follow-up is needed for several years after treatment to detect recurrence.

Key references
1. Binder H, Eng GD, Gaiser JF, et al.: Congenital muscular torticollis: results of conservative management with long term follow-up in 85 cases. Arch Phys Med Rehabil 1987, 68:222.
2. Canale ST, Griffin DW, Hubbard CN: Congenital muscular torticollis: a long term follow-up. J Bone Joint Surg [Am] 1982, 64:810.
3. Ferkel RD, Westin GW, Dawson ED, et al.: Muscular torticollis: a modified surgical approach. J Bone Joint Surg [Am] 1983, 65:894.
4. Phillips WA, Hensinger RN: The management of rotatory atlanto-axial subluxation in children. J Bone Joint Surg [Am] 1989, 71:664.

Diagnosis

History

Pain over the first annular pulley in the palm.

Finger may lock in flexion and often cannot be extended.

Symptoms usually worse in the morning and at the proximal interphalangeal joint.

Condition can affect the thumb and all digits.

Physical findings

Tenderness over the first annular pulley (Fig. 1).

Active demonstration of triggering (Fig. 2).

Fullness in the flexor tendon sheath.

Palpable nodule in the tendon sheath.

Imaging and laboratory studies

Radiography of involved digit to see whether there is a mechanical block in the joint.

Complications

Infection.

Digital nerve or vessel injury.

Painful scar.

Reflex sympathetic dystrophy.

Differential diagnosis

Volar retinacular cyst at first annular pulley.

Cystic degeneration in flexor tendons.

Mechanical locking due to osteophyte at proximal interphalangeal joint.

Etiology or pathophysiology.

Discrepancy in the size of the flexor tendon relative to the pulley of the fibrous flexor sheath.

Occasionally, people with amyloidosis will develop trigger finger.

Epidemiology

Usually occurs in middle-aged adults but can also occur in infants.

Women are more commonly affected.

Commonly seen in diabetic patients and patients with rheumatoid arthritis.

Multiple digits can be affected.

Associated with carpal tunnel syndrome and de Quervain's syndrome.

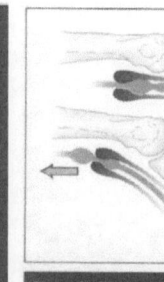

Figure 1. Stenosing tenosynovitis of the first annular pulley can result in a trigger finger involving any digit of the hand. The symptoms include locking of the finger in flexion and inability to fully extend the finger.

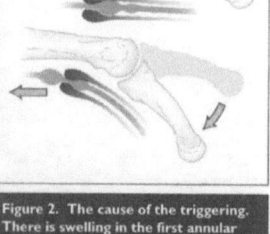

Figure 2. The cause of the triggering. There is swelling in the first annular pulley of the flexor tendon sheath, creating some nodularity in the flexor tendon itself. The stronger digital flexors enable flexion of the finger; the weaker digital extensors do not allow extension of the finger with the triggering phenomena.

Treatment

Nonsurgical

Nonsteroidal anti-inflammatory drugs may relieve symptoms but rarely correct the problem.

Steroid injections into the sheath temporarily help 60% to 80% of patients and may alleviate pain entirely.

Wrist splinting may help alleviate symptoms.

Surgical

Surgical release of the first annular pulley is effective in alleviating the problem in most cases.

Treatment aims
To prevent triggering phenomenon.
To prevent any significant attenuation of the tendon.
Often, if untreated, this condition can lead to reflex sympathetic dystrophy.

Prognosis
Surgery is almost 100% successful, and complications of pain, scarring, and reflex sympathetic dystrophy are infrequent.

Follow-up and management
The patient is initially placed in a bulky hand dressing and encouraged to flex and extend the digit actively. After the dressing is removed, the wound is kept dry for 2 weeks, then the sutures are removed. The scar is massaged with cream, which tends to soften the scar tissue.

Key references

1. Conklin JE, White WL. Stenosing tenosynovitis and its possible relation to the carpal tunnel syndrome. *Surg Clin North Am* 1960, 40:531–540.

2. Fahey JJ, Bollinger JA: Trigger finger in adults and children. *J Bone Joint Surg* 1954, 36A:1200–1218.

3. Lapidus PW: Stenosing tenovaginitis. *Surg Clin North Am* 1953, 33:1317–1347.

4. Medl WT: Tendonitis, tenosynovitis, "trigger finger" and de Quervain's disease. *Orthop Clin North Am* 1970, 1:373–382.

Diagnosis

Physical findings

Pain usually on the dorsum of the wrist or volarly near radial artery.

Swelling over the site of the ganglion (Fig. 1).

Feeling of fullness in the wrist.

Signs of nerve compression if ganglion is in carpal tunnel.

Cystic mass over dorsum of wrist or volarly near radial artery.

Cystic mass dorsally accentuated by wrist volar flexion.

Tenderness over origin of ganglion.

"Snapping" of tendons over the mass.

Imaging and laboratory studies

Radiography may reveal osteoarthritis in the wrist or cystic lesions in carpus.

Magnetic resonance imaging can differentiate ganglion from more serious masses.

Aspiration of mass reveals clear gelatinous fluid.

Differential diagnosis

Carpal boss.

Dorsal synovitis.

Traumatic.

Aneurysm.

Malignant tumor.

Etiology or pathophysiology

Possible herniation of wrist capsule.

Epidemiology

Peak incidence in young adults.

Slight female preponderance.

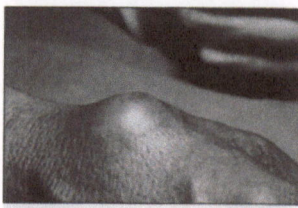

Figure 1. Dorsal wrist ganglions commonly occur along the radial aspect of the wrist, with swelling developing radially over the base of the index and thumb metacarpals. They are usually not pulsatile, are not fixed to the skin, and are transilluminated with a pin light. These ganglions usually arise from the scapholunate joint at the radial side of the wrist.

Treatment

Nonsurgical
Nonsteroidal anti-inflammatory drugs may decrease the pain and inflammation but usually do not cause disappearance of ganglion.

Aspiration and injection of the cyst with steroids are associated with a high recurrence rate.

Surgical
Surgical excision of the cyst with a portion of the capsule is usually successful.

Exercise and activity modification
No special precautions.

Prognosis
With surgical excision of the ganglion, recurrence rate is low.

Key references

1. Angelides AC, Wallace PF: The dorsal ganglion of the wrist: its pathogenesis, gross and microscopic anatomy, and surgical treatment. *J Hand Surg [Am]* 1976, 1:228–235.

2. Barnes WE, Larsen RD, Posch JL: Review of ganglia of the hand and wrist, with analysis of surgical treatment. *Plast Reconstr Surg* 1964, 34:570–578.

INDEX

Cefazolin
  for osteomyelitis, 141
  for septic arthritis, 167
Cefuroxime
  for osteomyelitis, 141
  for septic arthritis, 167
Celecoxib (Celebrex)
  adverse effects of, 124
  dosages of, 125
Celestone Soluspan
  for Baker's cyst, 17
  for impingement syndrome, 97
  for Morton's interdigital neuroma, 123
  for plantar fasciitis, 149
Cephalosporin
  for diskitis, 57
  for flexor tenosynovitis, 79
  for osteomyelitis, 141
Cervical collar, 37
Cervical fusion, 157
Cervical radiculopathy
  diagnosis of, 34
  differential diagnosis of, 34
  epidemiology of, 34
  etiology and pathophysiology of, 34
  history of, 34
  imaging and laboratory studies for, 34
  physical findings in, 34
  prognosis for, 35
  treatment of, 35
Cervical spine fractures
  classification of, 38
  complications of, 36
  CT scans of, 38–39
  diagnosis of, 36
  differential diagnosis of, 36
  epidemiology of, 36, 38
  etiology and pathophysiology of, 36
  follow-up and management of, 37
  history of, 36
  imaging and laboratory studies for, 36
  physical findings in, 36
  prognosis for, 37
  radiographs of, 38
  treatment of, 37–39
Cervical spondylosis
  diagnosis of, 40
  differential diagnosis of, 40
  epidemiology of, 40
  etiology and pathophysiology of, 40
  history of, 40
  imaging and laboratory studies in, 40
  physical findings in, 40
  prognosis for, 41
  treatment of, 41
  complications of, 40
Charcot arthropathy, 30
Cheilectomy, 105
Child abuse
  complications of, 42
  diagnosis of, 42
  differential diagnosis of, 42
  epidemiology of, 42
  etiology of, 42
  follow-up and management of, 43
  history of, 42
  imaging and laboratory studies for, 42
  physical findings in, 42
  prognosis for, 43
  treatment of, 43
Child protective services, 43
Children, back pain in, 14–15

Chondral replacement, 135
Chondrocalcinosis, 30
Chondroitin sulfate, 135, 139
Clavicle fractures
  complications of, 44
  diagnosis of, 44
  differential diagnosis of, 44
  epidemiology of, 44
  etiology and pathophysiology of, 44
  follow-up and management of, 45
  history of, 44
  imaging and laboratory studies in, 44
  physical findings in, 44
  prognosis for, 45
  treatment of, 45
Clawtoe deformity, 110
Clostridium flexor tenosynovitis, 78
Cobb angle, 164
Colchicine, 31, 89
Cold therapy See *also* Ice therapy
  for impingement syndrome, 97
  for rotator cuff tears, 159
Compartment syndromes
  with distal radius fractures, 62
  with intoeing surgery, 101
  treatment of, 63
Complete blood count
  for fingertip infection, 74
  for flexor tenosynovitis, 78
  for osteomyelitis, 140
Compression flexion injury, 37
Compression fractures
  cervical orthosis for, 37
  thoracolumbar, 182
Compressive dressing, 129
Compressive syndromes, 46–47 See *also* Cubital tunnel syndrome
Computed tomographic myelography, 40
Computed tomography
  for ankle fracture, 8
  for back pain in children, 14
  for cervical radiculopathy, 34
  for cervical spine fractures, 36, 38–39
  for child abuse, 42
  for comminuted fracture, 130
  coronal section, 130
  for degenerative lumbar disk disease and sciatica, 48
  for distal humerus fractures, 60
  for femoral shaft fractures, 72
  for flatfoot deformity, 76
  for hip dislocation, 58, 59
  indications for, 130
  for low back pain, 106
  principles of, 130
  for scaphoid fractures, 160
  for scoliosis, 164
  for seronegative spondyloarthropathy, 168
  for spinal stenosis, 172
  for spondylolisthesis, 174
  for tarsal coalitions, 180
  for thoracolumbar fractures, 182
  for tibial shaft fractures, 184
Conservative therapy
  for bipartite patella, 21
  for epicondylitis, 69
  for ingrown toenail, 99
Consultations, child abuse, 42
Core decompression, 143
Corns
  in metatarsalgia, 118
  treatment of, 119
  trimming of, 93
Corpectomy, anterior, 37

INDEX

INDEX

INDEX

INDEX

Vertebrae (*Continued*)
  tumors of, 164
Vertebral body
  destruction of, 56
  wedging of in Scheuermann's disease, *162*
Vertical compression fractures, 37
Vital signs, 182
Vitamin D, 145
Volar splint
  for carpal tunnel syndrome, 33
  for mallet finger, 109
Volkmann's ischemic contracture, 94

W

Warfarin
  displacement of, 124
  drug interactions of, 124
Warm compress, 129
Wartenberg's sign, 46
Water therapy, 157
Weakness, cervical, 34
Weight loss
  for low back pain, 107
  for osteoarthritis, 135
  for osteoarthritis of hip, 139
  for spinal stenosis, 173
Weight-bearing exercise

after bunion surgery, 27
after hip fracture, 81
for ankle fracture, 9
for femoral shaft fractures, 73
in hip dislocation, 59
with lateral ankle sprain, 102
for medial collateral ligament tears, 113
for metatarsal fractures, 117
for metatarsalgia, 119
in osteonecrosis, 143
for tibial shaft fractures, 185
Weight-bearing joints, degeneration of, 30
Weight-bearing pressure, 55
Wire fixation, 161
Wrist
  dorsoradial pain in, 50
  ganglion of, 84, 190–191
  immobilization of, 161
  splinting of, 189

X

Xanthine oxidase inhibitor, 89
X-ray absorptiometry, 144, *145*
Xylocaine
  for metatarsalgia, 118
  for Morton's interdigital neuroma, 122, 123
  for plantar fasciitis, 149